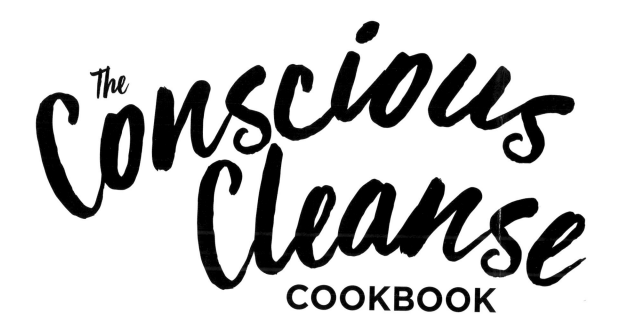

The Conscious Cleanse
COOKBOOK

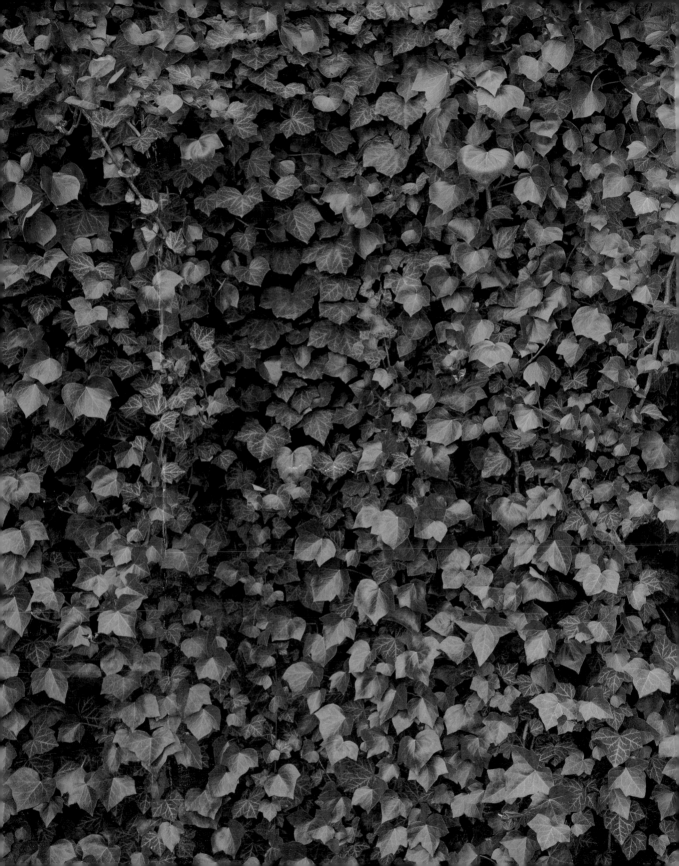

The Conscious Cleanse COOKBOOK

Julie Peláez & Jo Schaalman

ALPHA

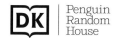

Publisher Mike Sanders
Editor Ann Barton
Book Designer Rebecca Batchelor
Photographer Daniel Showalter
Food Stylist Lovoni Walker
Proofreader Lisa Starnes
Indexer Celia McCoy
Recipe Testers Irena Shnayder and Trish Sebben Malone

First American Edition, 2020
Published in the United States by DK Publishing
6081 E. 82nd Street, Indianapolis, IN 46250

Library of Congress Catalog Number: 2020931143
ISBN: 978-1-4654-9332-3

DK books are available at special discounts when purchased
in bulk for sales promotions, premiums, fund-raising,
or educational use. For details, contact:
SpecialSales@dk.com

Printed and bound in Canada

Illustrations by Martha Daley
Cover image and pages 9, 12, 24, 29, 255 © Julia Vandenoever
All other images © Dorling Kindersley Limited

For the curious

www.dk.com

Dedicated to all who seek vibrant health.

May you always remember the value of infusing the food you cook with love.

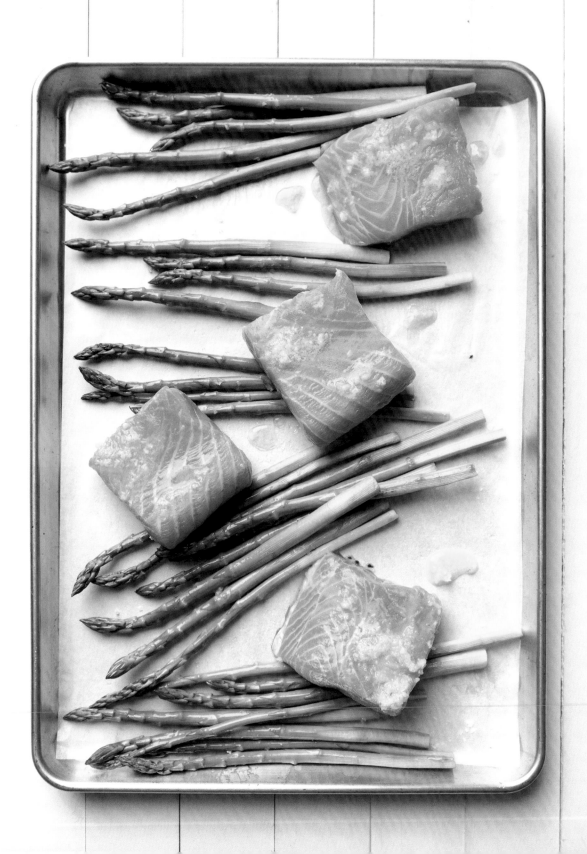

contents

INTRODUCTION 8

CONSCIOUS CLEANSE BASICS 11

GETTING STARTED 31

SMOOTHIES & JUICES 41

BREAKFASTS 63

SALADS.. 81

SOUPS.. 107

MEAT & SEAFOOD... 125

VEGETABLES 155

DIPS, SNACKS & STARTERS 179

SWEET TREATS 201

BEVERAGES & ELIXIRS 229

CONDIMENTS 241

RESOURCES 248

INDEX...252

introduction

Hey, there! We're Jo and Jules, the cofounders of the Conscious Cleanse. If you're like us, you've probably read more than your fair share of diet books. You likely have a kitchen cabinet full of beautiful cookbooks that you've hardly cracked—ones you purchased hoping for weight loss, glowing skin, more energy, and less pain. But alas, here you are, feeling subpar, while the cookbooks sit and collect dust.

Well, we have good news for you! You don't need another diet! And after devouring this cookbook, you won't need another cookbook either. You may want one for ideas and inspiration, but you won't need it.

When we created the Conscious Cleanse nearly 10 years ago, our goals were to teach people about getting back to the basics of eating real food and to help them identify food allergies and sensitivities, ultimately empowering them to become their best selves. After leading tens of thousands of people through our program, we know that it works. We also know that the single most powerful skill you can learn when it comes to taking charge of your health and making a sustainable lifestyle change is learning to make simple, nutrient-dense, home-cooked meals.

Our goal with *The Conscious Cleanse Cookbook* is simple—to get you in the kitchen, experimenting, cooking, chopping, peeling, tossing, grilling, and baking! Notice we put "experimenting" first. We want you to approach the recipes in this cookbook like an experiment: be curious, have fun, and above all else, forget the notion that every meal has to be a masterpiece. Once you start trying the recipes, you'll be pleasantly surprised to find that making healthy food can be both simple and delicious. Amazing things happen when you stock your kitchen with high-quality ingredients and cook with fresh produce. So, let go of the idea that you have to be perfect, dig in and get your hands dirty, and trust that you are in the right place.

No matter how many times you've found yourself grabbing a quick lunch from the drive-thru, shoveling in the kids' leftovers, or taking down a pint of ice cream, there is another way forward—one that's ripe with hope and possibility, and one that won't require you to spend all day in the kitchen. We know you're busy and have a lot of demands on your time. We get it! That's why the majority of the recipes in this book are quick and easy, without sacrificing flavor and nutrition.

Are you ready to get started? Are you ready to experience the wonders and the joys of vibrant health? We're so glad you're here, and we can't wait for you to dive into the recipes. If you have any questions or feedback at all, we would love to hear from you. Email us at joandjules@consciouscleanse.com or visit our website, consciouscleanse.com, for lots of free resources and access to our amazing online membership community.

With love from our kitchens to yours,
Jo and Jules

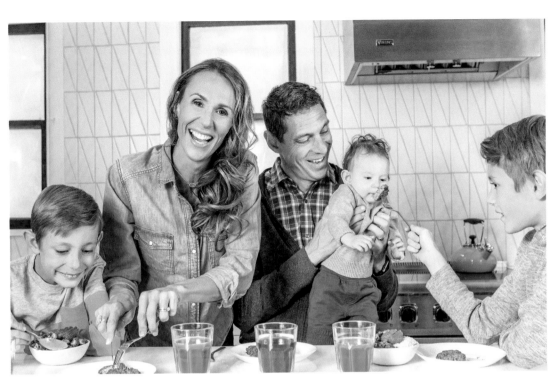
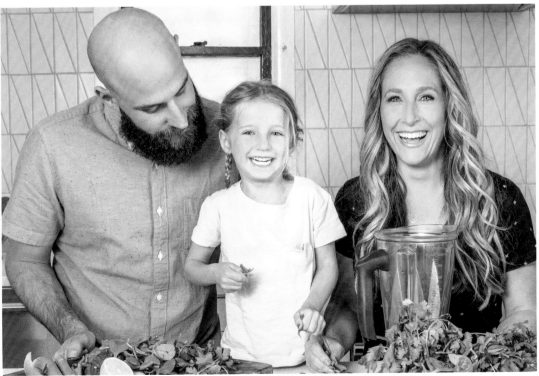

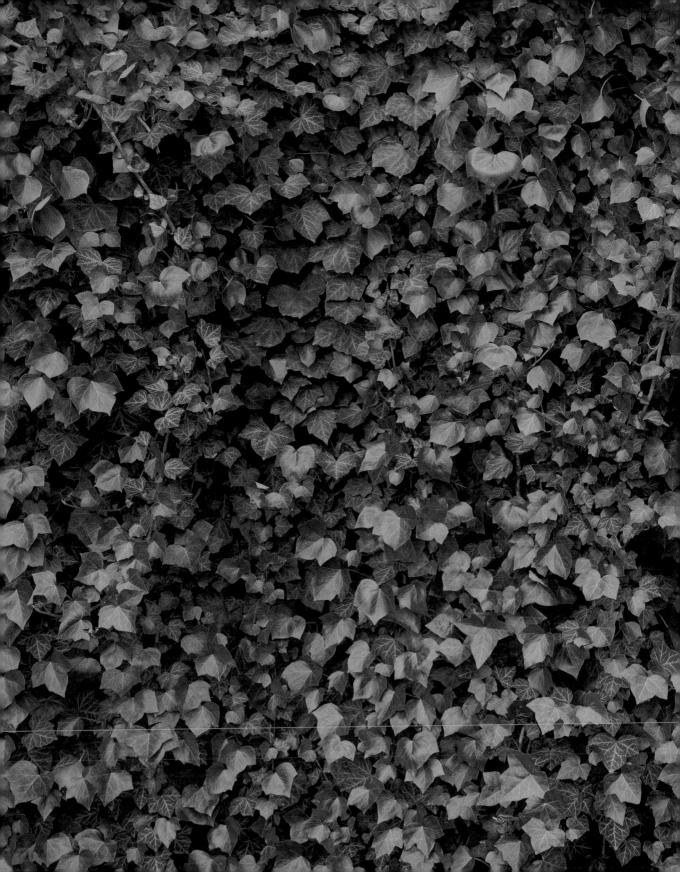

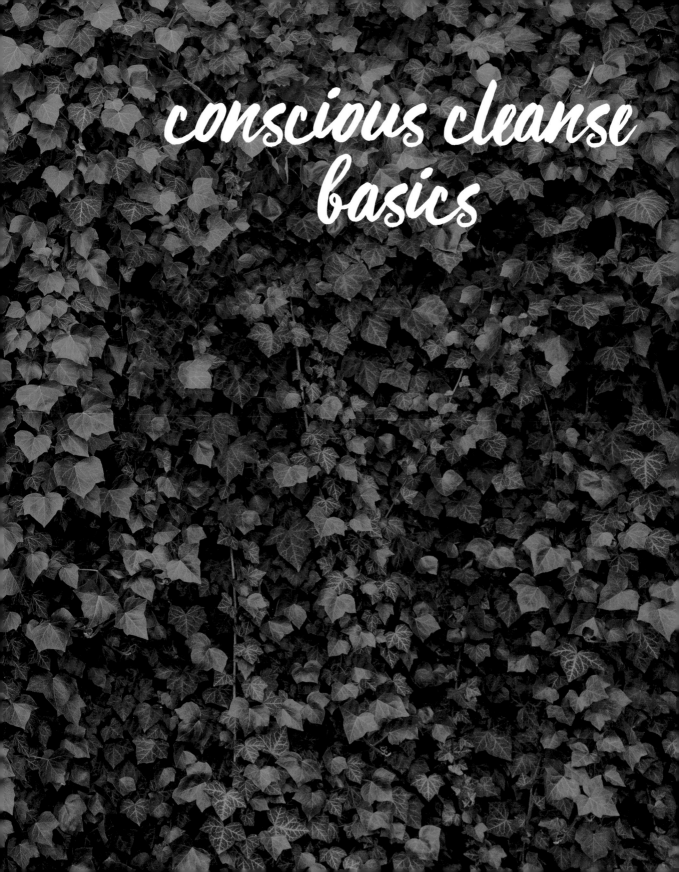

conscious cleanse basics

the conscious cleanse story

The Conscious Cleanse is not a diet. And we would argue that the last thing you need is another diet. What we all need (and truly want!) is the freedom and ease that come from living in a body that's free of nagging symptoms. We want to feel our best so we can show up for the ones we love and do the things we love to do. If you're ready to reclaim your health and vitality, you are in the right place!

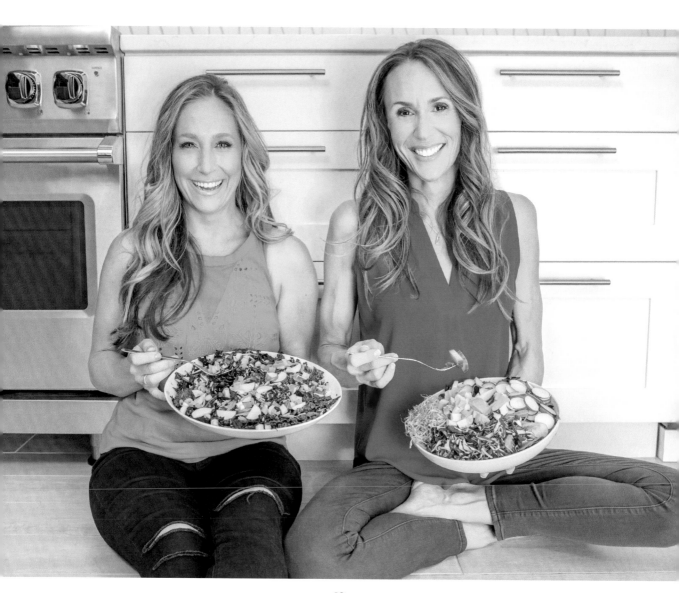

A SHARED PASSION

Back in 2010, we were going about our lives, independently teaching yoga and studying nutrition. For Jo, it was a terrible bike accident, where she broke her back, that brought her to look at food as medicine. She used both yoga and food to heal her debilitating chronic pain, in the process discovering how at odds she had been with her body her entire life. She realized from her accident that hope is the strongest medicine, and that's what we hope to provide everyone who joins our program. For Jules, it was sheer passion that called her to follow her heart into teaching yoga and studying nutrition. For all intents and purposes, she was a pretty darn healthy human—or so she thought.

We had no idea when we got together to test out some of the theories we'd been exploring independently that we would wind up developing a program that would help tens of thousands of people. Like a magical chance encounter, our parallel journeys ignited a shared passion to get the word out, on a global level: to help people access vibrant health, discover hidden food sensitivities, and completely rewire their brains about diets and "health" food.

AN INDIVIDUALIZED APPROACH

Drawing from each other's experiences helped us assemble the pieces of our own puzzles. In the process, we also realized what would become one of the core principles of the Conscious Cleanse—no two people are the same. Our bodies are intricate pulses of energies, each one unique in countless ways. And yet, the diet industry tries to convince us that we should all eat the exact same way. We're perfect examples of how important a bio-individualized approach to health and diet truly is. We came together from the opposite sides of the health spectrum, and our food preferences were just

as opposite. Jules is tall. Jo is short. Jules is brunette. Jo is blonde. Jules is long and lean. Jo is muscular. Jules doesn't eat meat. Jo does. Jules eats grains. Jo does not. For many years, we've joked that we're the yin and the yang, or the odd couple. But even in our wildest differences, we share deep commonalities. We personally found vibrant health and healing using similar overarching principles, but we individualized our approaches for our bodies, our own unique chemical makeups. And therein lies the power of the Conscious Cleanse philosophy.

A BLUEPRINT FOR SUCCESS

The Conscious Cleanse is a 14-day whole foods–based cleanse with a menu that includes delicious green smoothies; fresh vegetables and fruits; non-gluten grains, like brown rice and quinoa; beans; nuts and seeds; wild-caught fish; and organic, grass-fed meats. We eliminate all the common allergens, including eggs, dairy, gluten, sugar, soy, shellfish, nightshades, caffeine, and alcohol. After the 14-day journey, we teach you how to systematically reintroduce foods so that you can "test" them in your own body. The Conscious Cleanse is not a quick fix, and it's not an all-or-nothing approach. It's not about willpower or doing things "right." It's about slowing down and tuning in to your body to learn how food makes you feel.

The 14-day journey of the Conscious Cleanse is a guide to designing your own path to vibrant health. There is no one-size-fits-all solution, but we do share a common foundation that you can customize to suit your needs, likes, and dislikes. The Conscious Cleanse is about inclusivity. This is not the cool kids table. All are welcome—vegans, vegetarians, paleo, pescatarians, omnivores, the sugar sensitive, the AIPers, the FODMAPers, the diabetics, and those of you on an elimination diet. Everyone can have success eating the Conscious Cleanse way.

get into the conscious cleanse mindset

A "conscious cleanse" is one during which you gain deeper and deeper self-awareness and personal insights, while simultaneously undertaking a gentle detoxification of your system. This profound combination is the number-one reason why the Conscious Cleanse is the last program you'll ever need. Our goal is to give you a framework that sets you up for optimal health and healing, extraordinary longevity, and vibrant health—for the rest of your life. While this may sound like a lofty goal, it works because of the Conscious Cleanse mindset. So please, leave behind your diet mentality and toss out your scale because there is no calorie restriction or any strict food rules to follow on the Conscious Cleanse. There is no starving or depriving yourself, either. But there are also no shortcuts to success. The work must be done, but with the right mindset, the work—as well as the results—can be joyful.

TAKE A DEEP BREATH

There's no better way to slow down and bring yourself into the present moment than by taking a deep breath. Breathe in. Breathe out. When you remember to breathe, you pause, and in the pause, you create an opening to start to notice how you feel in your body. Let's give it a try, shall we? Breathe in ... how do you feel in your body right now? Breathe out ... what part of your body is calling or speaking to you? Is it your stomach, your lower back, your throat, your head? Your body communicates with you through signs, symptoms, and sensations. Tension is a great teacher. Your pain is the path. Take another deep breath, close your eyes, and, just for a moment, tune in, and listen to the wisdom that your body holds.

FOCUS ON WHAT YOU CAN EAT

The Conscious Cleanse includes an abundance of foods. Fresh fruits, like apples, pears, and blueberries. Nonstarchy vegetables, like cucumbers, carrots, broccoli, sprouts, and beets. Dark leafy greens, like spinach, romaine, arugula, and kale. Healthy fats, like olives, avocados, and cold-pressed olive oil. The list goes on—raw nuts and seeds; beans and legumes; starchy vegetables, like sweet potatoes and butternut squash; nongluten grains, like quinoa and brown rice; wild-caught fish; and organic, grass-fed meats, including bison and lamb. When you find yourself mentally stewing or obsessing over foods that are not on the Conscious Cleanse, gently bring your focus and attention back to the foods you can eat.

> With the Conscious Cleanse, I felt a whole shift in my mindset. Suddenly I was empowered to define my choices around food, my body, and how I would feel. I also discovered some nagging food allergies that had been making me feel tired and sluggish. After two weeks on the cleanse, I felt restored on a cellular level. I had no idea my body could feel this good, and I knew I could never go back.
> —Kate, Conscious Cleanser

DITCH THE WAGON

Have you ever uttered the words, "Ugh, I've fallen off the wagon," or "I've got to get back on the wagon"? This is an old mentality that must let go of if you are going to free yourself from yo-yo dieting. Ditching the wagon means that you learn from your so-called "slip-ups" when they happen without adding any extra guilt or shame. It means that if you happen to have a few bites of Ben & Jerry's ice cream, you catch yourself in the moment, acknowledge it, take a deep breath, and get curious about what else might be going on. Are you feeling overwhelmed, stressed, sad, lonely, or simply tired? Pre-Conscious Cleanse, you may have eaten the whole pint, telling yourself, "Screw it, I'll start over tomorrow." This is the cycle of guilt and shame that many of us have learned to overcome. The truth is, you don't need to start over tomorrow. Just make a better choice next time if need be. You've got this!

GET CURIOUS

Ready to take a deep dive into self-inquiry? It's time to take off the blinders and become an active participant in your own healing journey. And make no mistake, we all have work to do. At the core of the Conscious Cleanse is the willingness to look at all the ways in which we block ourselves from attaining what we say we want. Before you eat or drink anything, take a slow, deep, centering breath, and ask your body, "Will this food help me feel more vibrant?" Listen from your heart for the answers. Get curious about how you eat, not just what you eat. Do you eat while scrolling through social media or while multitasking? Once you are finished eating, tune into your body again. If you feel energized and gas-free, you're on the right track. On the other hand, if you feel tired or gassy, or develop a headache or a stomachache, those are signs that the food you ate (or the way in which you consumed it) was not ideal for you.

conscious cleanse guidelines

In a world of mixed dietary messages, fledgling nutrition science, and countless fad diets, it can feel nearly impossible to know what to eat anymore. Among all this chaos is the call to get back to the basics. The Conscious Cleanse answers that call with a return to simplicity. The following is a bird's-eye view of what to eat on the Conscious Cleanse. Combine these with the Conscious Cleanse mindset, and you'll be well on your way to reconnecting with the thriving, radiant, vibrant you!

EAT WHOLE FOODS

Whole foods are foods that exist in nature. Start by imagining a food's origins. Does it come from a living thing? Can you imagine it growing in a field, on a tree or bush, or in the ocean? Whole foods are foods that do not have ingredients—they are the ingredient. Whole foods are unprocessed, contain no hidden ingredients, and typically don't come in a package or have a label for you to examine. They often exist on the periphery of the grocery store, and they are colorful foods that fill farmers markets. Brown rice is a good example of a whole food, while rice cakes and brown rice pasta are not because they are more processed forms of the original. Whole foods include fresh fruit and vegetables, nongluten grains, legumes and beans, raw nuts and seeds, organic lean meats, and wild-caught fish.

—— WHOLE FOOD IMPOSTERS ——

Some processed foods may try to trick you into thinking they're whole foods, but they're not.

- Apple chips
- Banana bread
- Deli meat
- Flavored water
- Fruit juice
- Fruit leather
- Plantain chips
- Protein shakes
- Rice cakes
- Rice pasta
- Veggie straws
- Yogurt raisins
- Zucchini bread

> I am blown away at how my body is embracing this cleanse. My bloating is gone, especially around my midsection and face. My achy joints in the morning are also gone. My skin is glowing. This cleanse has been so easy to follow.
> —Silvia, Conscious Cleanser

ELIMINATE ALLERGENS

The Conscious Cleanse eliminates the most common food allergens. Some of these foods—like tomatoes, oranges, and eggs—may seem counterintuitive at first. But the fact is, it's estimated that up to 90 percent (stop and let that sink in) of Americans suffer from food intolerances or allergies, and most are undetected. That bears repeating. A whopping 9 out of 10 people may have some form of food intolerance, and most people do not make the link between the food they're eating and the physical ailments they're experiencing. If you've ever experienced any of the following, it's highly likely there is a food intolerance at play: bloating, cramps, diarrhea, constipation, headaches, dark circles under the eyes, clogged sinuses, puffiness, aches, pains, the inability to lose weight despite exercise and a "clean" diet, diabetes, high blood pressure, seasonal allergies, depression, or anxiety.

We know that giving up some of your favorite foods is challenging. We also know the rewards are worth it. Stop yourself if you start to get into a battle over a certain food, and remember it's often the foods we love and crave the most—the foods we're addicted to—that we benefit taking a break from the most. The good news is that at the end of 14 days, you'll be given a unique opportunity to do a mini-experiment with yourself, to isolate your favorite foods in a "clean" system, taking note of exactly how each one feels in your body. You're bound to learn something new about yourself and the food you eat!

FOODS TO KEEP OFF YOUR PLATE

- Alcohol
- Beef
- Caffeine
- Chocolate (cocoa and raw cacao included)
- Corn
- Dairy (cheese, yogurt, milk, whey protein, and butter)
- Eggs
- Grapefruit
- Nightshades (potatoes, tomatoes, eggplant, and peppers)
- Oranges
- Peanuts
- Pork
- Refined seed and vegetable oils (soy oil, sunflower oil, safflower oil, canola oil, corn oil, cottonseed oil)
- Shellfish (clams, crab, mussels, oysters, shrimp)
- Soy products (edamame, miso, tamari, tempeh, and tofu)
- Strawberries
- Sugar
- Wheat and gluten
- Yeast (including yeasted products like brewer's yeast and kombucha)

SUPPLEMENTS AND MEDICINES

We're often asked about supplements and medications on the Conscious Cleanse. First and foremost, always check with your medical provider before going off any prescribed medications or supplements. As a general rule of thumb, though, we like to occasionally eliminate all supplements in order to give our bodies a break. This is also a good time to take inventory. Make sure you know exactly what's in the supplements you're taking (pull out the magnifying glass and read the label), and re-evaluate whether those supplements still make sense for you. We also highly recommend that you avoid any over-the-counter drugs, such as painkillers or NSAIDs, as the daily use of such medicines has been linked to many dangerous side effects, the least of which is damaging the gastrointestinal tract. Tobacco, cannabis (marijuana), and street drugs are also not on the menu of the Conscious Cleanse.

GO PLANT POWERED

While most diet plans focus on food labels, which identify you as part of some type of "food club," we like to think that we're the program for all types of eaters. So, whether you'd call yourself paleo, pescatarian, omnivore, vegetarian, or vegan, all are welcome here. And frankly, we're less interested in what you call yourself and more interested in how many veggies you can fit on your plate.

Being plant-based is all the rage, but we have a newsflash for you—you don't have to be vegetarian or vegan to be plant-based. And guess what? You can eat meat and be plant-based, which is the best way to incorporate animal protein into your diet anyway. So, forget the food labels, and go plant powered with us! As far as how you eat your veggies, the sky's the limit, and this is where it gets fun! We love coming up with new ways to incorporate veggies into dishes and meals where you may not expect them. For example, a simple green smoothie can deliver an additional 2 cups of dark leafy greens with breakfast! Compare that to a typical breakfast, like a bagel with cream cheese, and you've got a massive breakfast makeover, one that's filled with bioavailable ingredients, alkaline-rich dark leafy greens, and an array of other nutrients and superfoods. This is just one way to add in more veggies, which can have a profound impact on your overall health.

We often recommend eating raw and living foods as much as possible because raw veggies have all their enzymes intact. Think of enzymes like the spark plugs of the body. Every single action in the body involves an enzymatic reaction, from blinking your eyes and wiggling your toes to digesting your food. Digestive enzymes help the body break down and assimilate the food you eat. So, the more enzymes you have, the better you're going to feel!

All that being said, there are some veggies, particularly cruciferous veggies like broccoli, cauliflower, and cabbage, that don't always sit well, gastrically speaking. If you find that you get a tummy ache, gas, or bloating after eating certain raw veggies,

—— HEAL THE GUT, HEAL THE BODY ——

Would it surprise you to learn that an unbalanced microbiome is the root cause of most chronic and degenerative illnesses? It's true! But taking a probiotic supplement is just part of the story. Supplementing your diet with foods rich in healthy probiotics, like our Vegan Kimchi (page 242), is key. You also want to eat good sources of prebiotics. Foods like artichokes, asparagus, bananas, chickpeas, dandelion greens, garlic, and onions actually feed beneficial bacteria in your gut. Eat a wide variety of different types of veggies, and not only will you be getting all the right nutrients, you'll also help balance the good and bad bugs in your gut.

This has been a great experiment that is becoming the new norm. We used to talk about dinner and say, "Where are we going?" Now we say, "Which recipe should we cook?" My husband and I are both down in weight and body fat, which is terrific. We like these changes so much, and it's been mostly easy! The recipes aren't difficult, and they are full of flavors.
—Holly, Conscious Cleanser

go ahead and cook them. We love our vegetables lightly steamed, sautéed, grilled, and/or roasted—all depending on the season and our mood. This is again where you can practice tuning in and asking yourself, "Will this food (and the way I prepare it) help me feel more vibrant?"

Finally, if you ever experience any constipation or diarrhea, cooking your veggies can be very helpful. These symptoms can be a sign of inflammation in the gut, perhaps from eating foods you're allergic to. Cooking your veggies may feel more soothing to your system as you clean it up and heal your gut.

EAT CLEAN FOODS

We've already defined whole foods as foods that exist in nature and have not been altered from their original state. Unfortunately, eating "clean" is not as easy or simple as choosing between broccoli and Cheez-Its. As with anything, shades of gray flank the black and white, so it's worth taking a closer look.

Clean foods are package-free foods. Many of our kitchen staples can be found in the bulk section of your local grocery or health food store—things like nongluten grains, beans, raw nuts and seeds, even spices, dried herbs, and dried fruit. The other mainstay of our eating plan is, as we've mentioned, fresh fruits and vegetables—again, no special or fancy packaging is necessary.

Where we often run into trouble with clean eating is with store-bought products that are mired in labels touting eye-catching marketing claims; gluten-free, soy-free, dairy-free, and non-GMO. It must be clean, right? We've found the worst culprits to be the dips, dressings, sauces, condiments, and nut milks—products that are supposed to make our clean eating journey easier. Sadly, we can't tell you how many times we've fallen into the trap of thinking a product is clean and "safe," only to bust out the magnifying glass and learn that sugar is the second ingredient. If you're going to buy a packaged food, be a label detective.

Focus on the list of ingredients in the food. A couple general rules of thumb are: the fewer the ingredients, the better, and if you can't pronounce it or have to ask someone what it is or does, skip it.

MAKE YOUR OWN STAPLES

The good news is that the cookbook you're holding in your hands is full of our favorite food makeovers, like Egg-Free Avocado Mayo (page 245) or Chocolate Dessert Hummus (page 212). These recipes were inspired by products we found in the store with ingredients that didn't match up to our standards. Other great examples are our Homemade Plant-Based Milks (pages 230–231). In fact, we only make our own oat milk because there is currently no gluten-free, organic option on the market. Once you learn how simple (and cost effective) it is to make some of your own staples, you'll never go back to premade ones.

DITCH PLASTICS

We've all heard about the harmful effects of bisphenol A (BPA), a chemical in plastics, on the human body, but once BPA-free products began hitting the grocery store shelves, many people let out a sigh of relief thinking that was the end of it. Sadly, that's not the case, and we are learning that we're inadvertently eating up to a credit card's worth of microplastics each week! Luckily, there are many things you can do to minimize consuming plastic. In addition to storing your food in glass containers whenever possible, not buying produce in plastic can make a huge difference. We know it's convenient to buy the tub of spinach or big bag of romaine lettuce, but avoiding these will help you reduce your plastic consumption while also helping the environment.

easy-in, easy-out food combinations

Would you believe us if we told you that digestion requires more energy than any other function in the human body? Experts agree that up to 80 percent of the body's energy goes to digesting the food we eat! Just think of how much energy you could free up if you learned to eat in a way that optimized digestion. Goodbye post-lunch nap, hello increased productivity!

Easy-in, easy-out food combining is one of the key components to success on the Conscious Cleanse. Perhaps the world's best-kept secret for ongoing weight loss and weight management, food combining helps improve digestion, thereby reducing the burden of digestion on the body.

Nearly 2,500 years ago, the ancient Greek physician Hippocrates said, "All disease begins in the gut." We like to think that health begins in the gut, which is why food combining is such an important part of the Conscious Cleanse and our 80:20 Plan. Although weight loss is a great side benefit of food combining, the real magic comes from a system that's free from excess gas, bloating, constipation, belching, and reflux. The result is better nutrient absorption and assimilation, making the healthy food you eat that much more powerful.

The only thing more important than what you eat is how well you digest it and eliminate it. On the Conscious Cleanse, you'll be eating fiber- and enzyme-rich food; food that is brimming with life-force energy; and food that is anti-inflammatory, alka-lizing, and hydrating. The real power in this food plan, however, is that it will attract and pull toxins from your tissues and cells, getting them ready for elimination. Food combining ensures that you get these toxins out of the body as quickly and efficiently as possible.

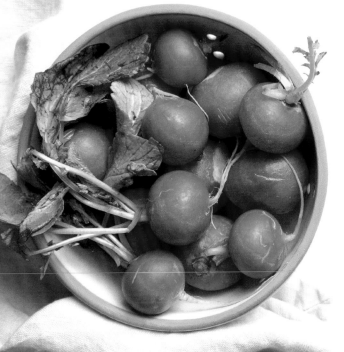

DON'T WORRY!

Although food combining can feel complicated and a little confusing to the uninitiated, we encourage you to give it a try! Keep it simple and remember, no two bodies are the same and each person's digestive system is unique. That said, forge ahead and let this be part of your cleanse experiment where ultimately, you get to make up your own "rules."

STEP 1: PICK ONE CATEGORY PER MEAL.

Animal Proteins

Bison

Lamb

Poultry

Seafood

Wild game

Starches

Beans and legumes (black beans, chickpeas/garbanzo beans, lentils)

Nongluten grains (brown rice, quinoa, millet)

Sweet potatoes

Winter squash (acorn, butternut, spaghetti)

Nuts / Seeds / Dried Fruit

Raw nuts (almonds, cashews, walnuts)

Raw seeds (sunflower, pumpkin, hemp, chia)

Dried fruits (unsulfured and unsweetened dried cranberries, figs, dates, raisins)

Fresh Fruits

Apples

Bananas

Berries

Cantaloupe

Grapes

Mangoes

Peaches

Pears

Pineapple

STEP 2: FILL THE REST OF YOUR PLATE WITH NONSTARCHY VEGGIES (NEUTRAL).

Artichokes

Arugula

Asparagus

Avocados

Beets and beet greens

Bok choy

Broccoli

Brussels sprouts

Cabbage

Carrots

Cauliflower

Chard

Collard greens

Cucumbers

Dandelion greens

Garlic

Ginger

Green beans

Kale

Leafy green herbs

Lettuce

Onions

Parsnips

Radishes

Spinach

Sprouts

Zucchini

STEP 3: WAIT BEFORE EATING AGAIN.

Wait 3 to 4 hours before switching to a different category. If you are hungry between meals, nonstarchy veggies (preferably raw) are always a safe bet.

Notes and Exceptions

Fruit is best eaten alone and on an empty stomach. Repeat: eat it alone or leave it alone. Most fruit takes about 30 minutes to digest.

Dried fruit is best on an empty stomach. Dried fruit takes longer than fresh fruit to digest, so apply the 3-hour rule here.

Avocado is technically a starch-combining "fruit," but we keep it in the neutral category since it's usually a garnish and not a prominent ingredient.

The following can be considered neutral: lemon juice, lime juice, olive oil, coconut milk, and nut milks.

Green smoothies are blended and therefore "predigested," making it okay to combine fruit and dark leafy greens, along with a nut milk or other boosts like hemp seeds or chia seeds.

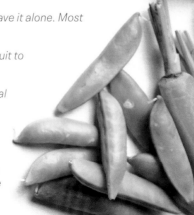

the conscious cleanse plate

We created the Conscious Cleanse Plate as a visual guide to a typical meal on the Conscious Cleanse. Two thirds of the plate is filled with nonstarchy vegetables, and the remaining one third comes from your choice of the following: animal protein, starch (nongluten grain or cooked starchy vegetable), beans, nuts, or seeds. Think of nonstarchy veggies as the center of your food universe, and you'll be on your way to reducing aches and pain in your body, slaying inflammation, healing your gut, and releasing extra weight.

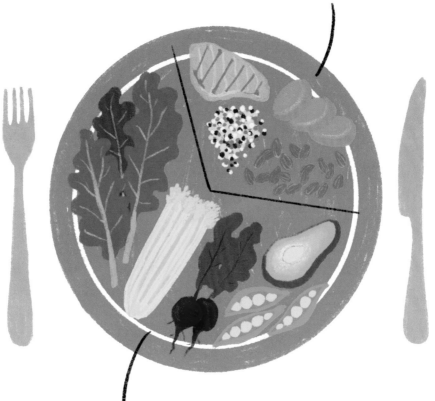

Add ⅓ animal protein, starch, beans, nuts, or seeds

fill your plate ⅔ with veggies

14-day conscious cleanse
AT–A–GLANCE

Wondering what you're going to eat on the 14-day Conscious Cleanse? Here is your at-a-glance guide!

- Start the day with 1 quart warm lemon water.

- When hungry, have 1 quart green smoothie as your first meal.

- At lunch and dinner, follow the Conscious Cleanse Plate. Eat unlimited nonstarchy veggies, plus your choice of an animal protein *or* a starch (nongluten grain or cooked starchy vegetable) *or* beans *or* nuts/seeds.

- Enjoy one to three servings of fresh fruit per day, as desired.

- Drink at least half your body weight in ounces of pure water. For example, if you weigh 150 pounds, you would drink 75 ounces of water.

- Snack between meals if hungry. (Just be mindful when switching food combining categories, and when in doubt, choose raw veggies.)

the 80:20 lifestyle plan

We have a confession. The Conscious Cleanse isn't really a 14-day program. And by the time you arrive at day 14, you'll understand why. When we developed the Conscious Cleanse we were clear on our mission—to help our participants create long-lasting, sustainable changes. Period. After the cleanse is over, you're a clean canvas, giving you a very unique opportunity upon which you can design a "food lifestyle" of your very own. Our 80:20 Lifestyle Plan gives you a framework for integrating what you learn from the Conscious Cleanse with the less-than-healthy foods you love and don't want to say goodbye to forever.

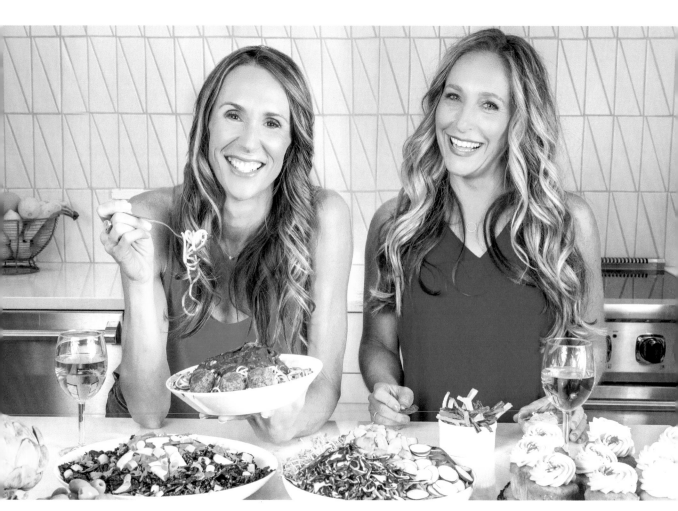

DOING THE ABCs

Long before "clean eating" became the catchphrase of the wellness world, we talked about cleansing as a lifestyle. We affectionately called this "doing the ABCs"—an acronym for "always be cleansing." Now, this in no way means that you should be on a formal cleanse year-round—far from it. It simply means that you can (and we dare say should) eat and live in a way that supports your body's natural ability to detoxify on an ongoing basis—and a way that optimizes digestion and promotes a healthy gut. In order to support our participants in doing their ABCs, we created our 80:20 Plan. Simply stated, the 80:20 is about following the Conscious Cleanse 80 percent of the time and throwing any notion of deprivation out the window the other 20 percent of the time.

Liberating, isn't it? Time for the happy dance? We think so! To sustain a lifelong path, you need to give yourself the freedom to stray from that path once in a while. You do this from a place of informed choice, from a place of empowerment, without guilt or regret, knowing exploration is a crucial part of the human spirit. But also be aware that straying too far can get you lost … and back to a long list of unwanted symptoms.

FOOD REINTRODUCTION

So, let's talk about informed choice on the 80:20 Plan. Although technically part of the Conscious Cleanse, it's important we mention the food reintroduction phase here because it's a crucial step in figuring out if you have food allergies or sensitivities. This will be the information you use to craft your personal 80:20 plan.

Using the clean slate that you create during the Conscious Cleanse, you will slowly reintroduce the foods that you kept off your plate during the cleanse and observe exactly how those foods make you feel. It's important to take it slowly and reintroduce one food at a time (one allergen per day while continuing to eat according to the Conscious Cleanse guidelines) to determine if the food is one that contributes to your overall energy and mental clarity, or on the contrary, makes you feel sluggish and bloated. In our first book, *The Conscious Cleanse,* and in our online program, we guide participants through this process in a very systematic way so you can really hone in on your reactions and results. This is all part of the personal experiment that is the Conscious Cleanse. Once you gather all of your data, you'll be able to map out a personalized 80:20 plan. We all have varying degrees of sensitivities, what we can and cannot "get away with," so it's going to be up to you to decide if you can (or want to) include the occasional piece of birthday cake or burger and fries in your 80:20 plan.

> Not only has the Conscious Cleanse helped me upgrade my diet, but I now know my sensitivity to dairy was more intense than I once thought. I've also gained mental clarity and have a clear path moving forward as I tackle healing my prostate, creating a clean relationship with food, and enjoying healthy lifestyle choices.
> —Greg, Conscious Cleanser

your 80:20 plan

The 80:20 isn't a one-size-fits-all plan. Much like the cleanse, this is an individualized process that's based on your unique blueprint, your health and fitness goals, and, ultimately, how you feel.

We've had many participants find success following the principles of the Conscious Cleanse on the weekdays and then letting it go for a few meals over the weekend. The 80 percent in this scenario would mean a cleanse-friendly breakfast and lunch on Friday and a 20 percent dinner, which might include a plate of cheesy Mexican food, corn tortilla chips, and a margarita (or two!). If you wake up Saturday feeling sluggish, it's right back to a green smoothie for breakfast, and ideally, a day of clean eating. Sunday morning, if you wake up feeling good and pancakes are on the menu, you may choose to go for it again!

The bottom line is that there is no hard-and-fast rule or way to piece together your personal 80:20 plan. Your body will let you know. If you stop releasing weight or have other symptoms resurface, it might be that your 80:20 has become a 60:40. Be honest with yourself. Stay aware. And continue to engage with the process. Sooner rather than later, you'll find what works for you and what you can "get away with" while still experiencing your ideal body weight, sound sleep, bright skin, and mental clarity.

THE 80 PERCENT

During your clean-eating (80 percent) time, you'll fix meals that abide by the Conscious Cleanse guidelines. Focus on eating whole foods. Eat in easy-in, easy-out food combinations. Start the day with warm water and lemon, followed by a green smoothie for your first meal. Use the Conscious Cleanse Plate as your guide, and fill your plate with at least two-thirds veggies and your choice of a protein, starch, beans, or nuts/seeds. Drink at least half your body weight in ounces of pure water. Do these things most days, and you'll have a really healthy foundation on which you can experiment during your 20 percent.

THE 20 PERCENT

It doesn't really matter when you choose to take your 20 percent time, as long as you do it consciously. It will likely come as no surprise that we suggest keeping sugar, gluten, and dairy out of your 80 percent zone. That being said, as long as you don't experience any severe reactions, just about anything goes during your 20 percent time without running the risk of overloading the body and its detoxification channels.

FOOD COMBINING ON THE 80:20

Once you get seasoned at practicing easy-in, easy-out food combining—and experience the benefits—you'll never go back. It's for this reason that food combining is part of our 80 percent. You might be wondering how to food combine a few of the foods that we kept off our plate during the Conscious Cleanse, such as dairy and eggs. So, here it goes: cheese, eggs, milk, and yogurt all combine like an animal protein. Remember, keep your meals simple and filled with veggies. Your digestive system will thank you.

DISCOVERING YOUR 80:20

We encourage you to take on defining and refining your 80:20 much like you did on the cleanse—with curiosity and joy. If you find your 80:20 does a 180, it's part of the exploratory process. You know what to do in order to get back to ground zero, where you're at (or moving toward) your ideal body weight, enjoying boundless energy, and feeling symptom-free.

You'll find that a funny thing happens as you follow the 80:20. If you pay attention to it, you'll notice that your cravings for "bad" stuff will begin to shift. All of a sudden, these foods don't taste as good as you remember. Indulgences become more refined, more intentional, and more mindful, and you don't need to "pull yourself back" the way you used to. In fact, you may just find yourself looking forward to getting back to your 80 percent as much as you look forward to your 20 percent. Balance is a beautiful thing indeed.

GOOD, BETTER, BEST

In our online membership program, we offer members a Good Better Best Guide as part of learning how to refine and up-level their choices in the 20 percent zone. Think of this like crossing over a bridge. Depending on your starting point, move from good to better to best as a way to experiment with a healthier variation. Foods in the Better and Best columns tend to be less inflammatory, less processed, and more nutrient dense.

Even though pretty much anything goes during the 20 percent time, we've found this to be a fun way to experiment with our diets. In other words, if there is a food or a dish that you absolutely love, can you upgrade some of the ingredients using a good, better, best approach? An easy one is sugar. Many baked goods call for white or brown sugar. You might be pleasantly surprised to discover just how delicious an alternative like monk fruit is. Not to mention that it has zero (yes, zero) calories and is known to alleviate inflammation and promote weight loss.

FOOD	GOOD	BETTER	BEST
White rice	Brown rice	Quinoa	Cauliflower rice
Cheese	Goat or sheep's milk cheese	Store-bought cashew or almond cheese	Homemade cashew feta
Refined white sugar or artificial sweeteners (Splenda, Equal, aspartame)	Brown rice or date syrup	Pure maple syrup or local honey	Stevia or monk fruit sweetener

80:20 guidelines
AT–A–GLANCE

Ready to dive into 80:20 living? Here's your guide to get started!

- Identify any food allergies or sensitivities to determine which foods you want to include in your 20 percent.

- Track your 80:20 meals for one week, along with any changes in how you're feeling. Adjust course as needed.

- Start the day with 1 quart warm lemon water.

- When hungry, have 1 quart green smoothie as your first meal.

- Keep a veggie-centric approach to every meal.

- Practice easy-in, easy-out food combining.

- Eat fruit alone, or leave it alone (except when blended).

- Drink at least half your body weight in ounces of pure water each day. For example, if you weigh 150 pounds, you would drink 75 ounces of water.

- Snack between meals if hungry. (Just be mindful when switching food-combining categories, and when in doubt, choose raw veggies.)

- Take one of your favorite splurges per week and try to up-level it with one of the recipes in this book. Got a thing for chocolate ice cream? Try our Chocolate Chickpea Ice Cream (page 226). We promise you won't be disappointed.

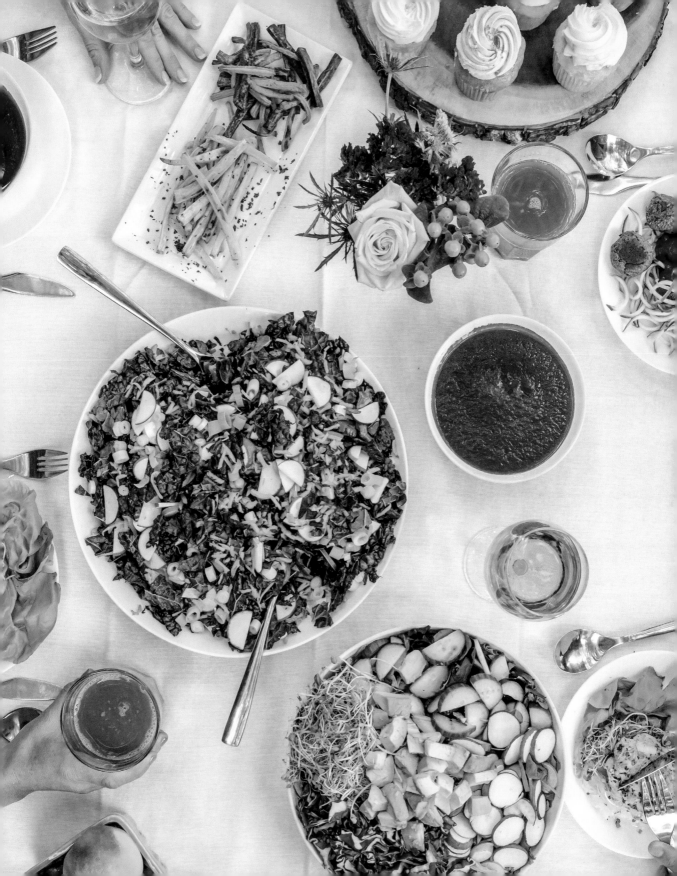

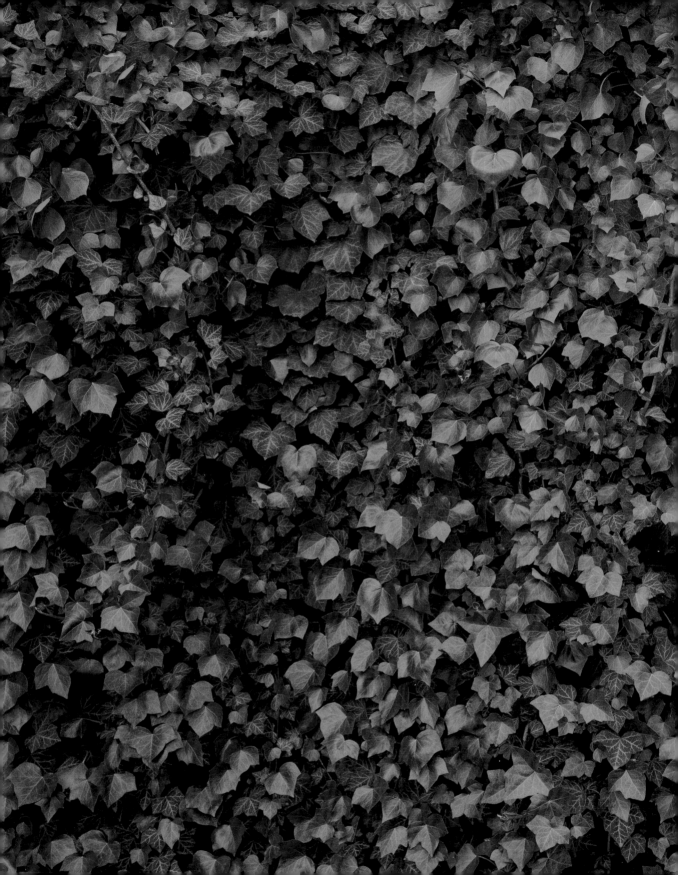

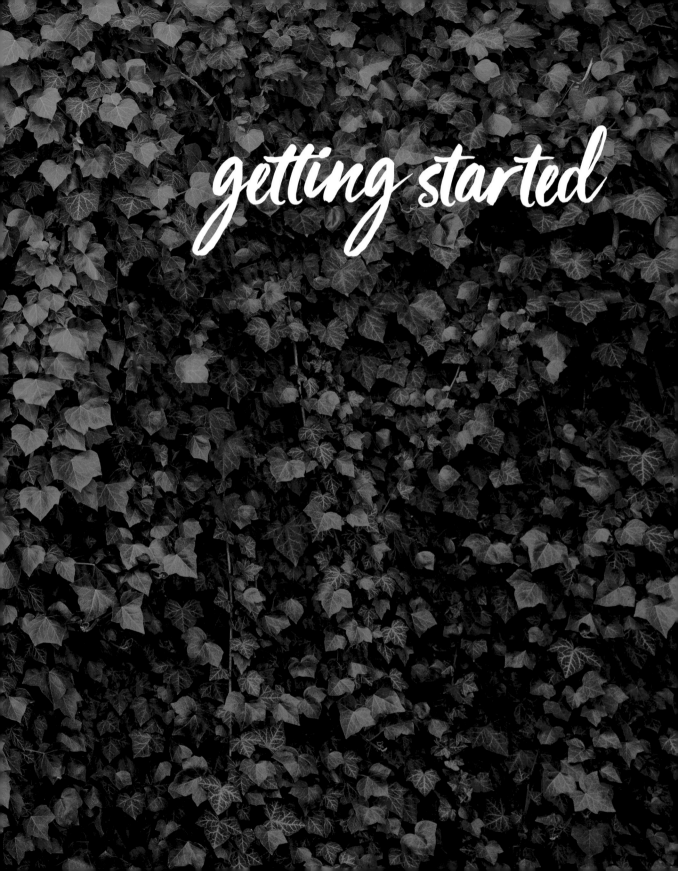

set yourself up for success

Planning and preparation are the keys to success on the Conscious Cleanse. Here are some simple steps to get you started right away. For a more detailed step-by-step plan for getting started on the cleanse, see Part 1 in our first book, *The Conscious Cleanse,* or visit our website, consciouscleanse.com, where we support a vibrant community of people like you in our online membership program.

CHOOSE A START DATE

Choosing a time to do the Conscious Cleanse is not as hard as it may seem. In fact, if you look at your calendar right now, you'll likely find an event, special occasion, or work trip that makes you think now is not the right time. Well, here's what we've learned for sure: you don't find time, you make it. And if you wait for the perfect time, you'll never start because it doesn't exist. The time is now. So, pull out your calendar and block off 14 days. And remember, in the big scheme of life, it's just 14 days.

Give yourself this gift, and while you're at it, really throw yourself into the process. Tell yourself, "This is an experiment I'm committed to. I'm going to step out of my comfort zone for the next two weeks. I can do anything for two weeks."

PREPARE FOR PURIFICATION

During the Conscious Cleanse, you'll have two opportunities to experience Purification. Days 6–7 and days 13–14 are times of rest where you'll eat exclusively fruits, vegetables, nourishing soups, juices, smoothies, and broth. This is optional, but encouraged, as it can be a profound healing experience. As we've mentioned, up to 80 percent of your body's energy goes to digestion. During Purification, you free up more of that energy, which equates to turning over new cells while resting and detoxing the other organs in the body like your kidneys and liver. It's crucial that you rest during Purification, so pull out your calendar again and clear away any unnecessary commitments.

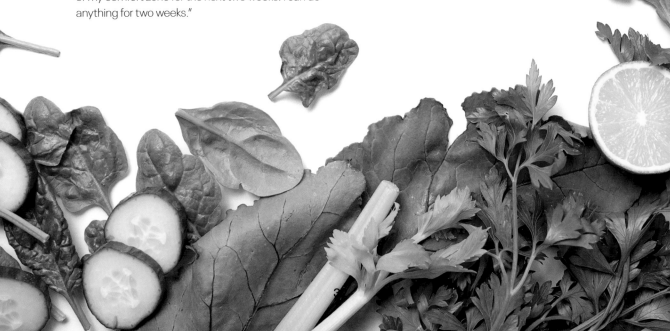

MAKE A PLAN

We repeat: you don't find time, you make it. Having a plan for tomorrow allows you to live in the moment today. Practically speaking, we suggest you finish reading this chapter before beginning your official cleanse. Get your kitchen ready; stock your pantry with the essentials; flip through the recipes; look over the sample meal plans; and write out a plan for your breakfast, lunch, and dinner for the first 3 to 5 days on the cleanse.

Next, take another look at your calendar and write down every possible tricky situation that might come up during the course of your cleanse. These may include a business lunch, a weekend getaway, a friend's birthday party, or feeding the family. Think through each one of these possible scenarios, and make a plan for how you will address them. We would even go so far as to say mentally rehearse it beforehand. We'll say it again: preparation is the key to success. Here are some examples of potentially tricky situations and our advice for how to handle them.

DINING OUT

The best advice we can give you about eating out in a restaurant is to ask for what you need. With a big smile, tell your server you're doing a food experiment and have some special requests. Take a look at the menu, and treat it like a list of ingredients. (It can be helpful to look at the menu online ahead of time whenever possible.) Build your own salad topped with some animal protein, and use olive oil and lemon for dressing. Simple.

EATING ON THE ROAD

Before you leave, scout out a local health food store and restaurants that offer a good variety of healthy options. Try to reserve a hotel room with a mini-fridge, or simply get a bucket of ice for any perishable items you buy when you arrive. Bring food with you. We call this our "conscious snack pack" and rarely leave home without it. Pack some water, carrots and celery sticks, and a small baggie of raw nuts or seeds. You might even make your own stir-fry before you leave and pack it in a reuseable container. While everyone else is busting out their fast food, you can sit back and enjoy your home-cooked meal. Don't forget to bring an extra avocado, an apple, some herbal tea, and stevia.

RECRUIT A BUDDY

Finding a cleanse buddy and creating a system of support around you is one of the best ways to set yourself up for success on the Conscious Cleanse. Not only is it rewarding to share your experiences with someone else, it's also super helpful to have a friend, family member, or housemate to share in the food shopping and preparation.

At the very least, share your intention and commitment with someone close to you. Explain why you're undertaking the experiment, and make it personal. Here's an example that you might share with your family: "I'm starting the 14-day Conscious Cleanse to see if changing my diet will help me sleep better and have more energy so I can be a better mom and wife. Anyone want to join me? I'm going to be trying some new recipes, and I'd love it if you'd try them with me."

CHOOSE YOUR TRACK

The Conscious Cleanse offers a baseline program that's fully customizable based on your individual needs. There's no such thing as "doing it right"; there's only "doing it right for you." With that in mind, we've created three different tracks as a guide for how to get started on the Conscious Cleanse. As with all good adventures, you'll benefit from side trips and experiments, but the tracks will give you a framework to begin. For more guidance, check out our meal plans in the Resources section (pages 250–251).

PLANT POWERED

Although not strictly a vegan plan, this track is for you if the idea of going without any animal protein is no big deal. If you're ready to embrace a diet that is 75 to 80 percent raw foods, but look forward to the grounding nature of cooked quinoa, roasted veggies, and the occasional serving of chickpeas or black beans, this track is for you. In addition to the large baseline of nonstarchy, water-containing, alkaline veggies, the Plant Powered Track includes some fruit, nongluten grains, raw nuts and seeds, beans, legumes, and natural sweeteners like maple syrup and honey.

MEAT LOVER

If you know your body craves animal protein or you've ever said, "I don't function until I've had some protein," then this is the track for you. You may have tried programs or diet plans in the past that are very meat heavy, but this plan is far from a free pass to eat bacon for breakfast, lunch, and dinner. What's different about the Meat Lover Track is the large volume of water-containing, alkaline veggies that are eaten alongside animal protein. Approved animal proteins include wild fish and seafood, organic poultry, and grass-fed meats, including bison and lamb.

LOW SUGAR

If you have intense sugar cravings or hormonal imbalances, or struggle to lose weight, or deal with blood sugar issues or insomnia, the Low Sugar Track is for you. What sets the Low Sugar Track apart from the others is a greater focus on protein and healthy fats while limiting grains and beans, natural sweeteners (like honey and maple syrup), and having only 1 cup of low-glycemic fruit per day. On the Conscious Cleanse, you'll eliminate all artificial and refined sugars completely, but if you think you have a sugar sensitivity or are ready to tame the sugar beast, this is the track for you.

TAKE OUR SUGAR SENSITIVITY QUIZ

Sugar is eight times as addictive as cocaine, so it's no wonder so many people struggle to give it up. Hidden sugar is in nearly all processed foods: yogurt, milk, crackers, peanut butter, salad dressings, and condiments, just to name a few. Sugar is at the root cause of many chronic health conditions such as obesity, diabetes, heart disease, cancer, acne, depression, anxiety, insomnia, and more. Think you're addicted to sugar? Take our Sugar Sensitivity Quiz at consciouscleanse.com/sugarquiz.

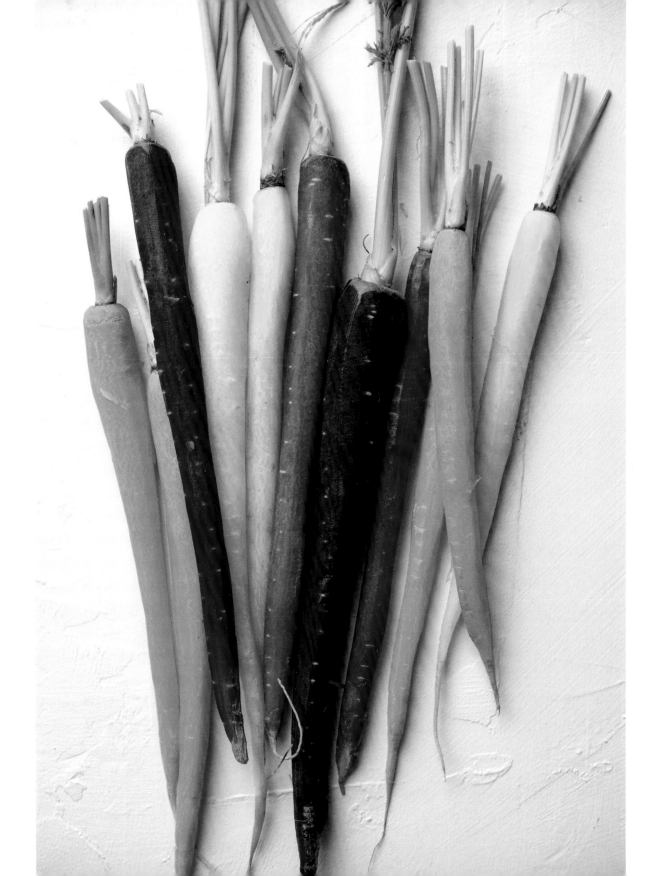

GET YOUR KITCHEN READY

One of the questions we hear a lot is, "Am I going to have to spend all day in the kitchen?" While there is definitely some kitchen time required, a little forethought goes a long way. Stocking your kitchen with essential gear and basic pantry items will help to make meal prep a simple and relatively unobtrusive task.

TOOLS

Cookware

Cutting board

Food processor

Glass storage containers

High-speed blender (we love Vitamix)

Juicer (we love Breville or Omega)

Mason jars

Mesh strainer

Nut milk bag

Peeler

Sharp knife

Slow cooker or multicooker (we love Instant Pot)

Spiralizer

Steamer basket

PANTRY STAPLES

These are some of the ingredients we always have stocked, whether cleansing or living the 80:20. Check out Brands We Love and Trust (page 249) for specific brand recommendations.

oils & vinegars

Avocado oil

Coconut oil

Olive oil

Toasted sesame oil

Apple cider vinegar

Brown rice vinegar

Red wine vinegar

Ume plum vinegar

Note: It's important to seek out high-quality oils; look for organic, unrefined, and cold pressed.

raw nuts & seeds

Almonds

Brazil nuts

Cashews

Chia seeds

Flaxseeds

Hazelnuts

Hemp seeds

Macadamia nuts

Pecans

Pine nuts

Pumpkin seeds

Sesame seeds (white and black)

Sunflower seeds

Walnuts

nut & seed butters

Raw almond butter

Raw tahini

Sunflower seed butter

Note: It's important to seek out high-quality nuts and seeds and their butter counterparts. Look for raw and organic whenever possible. Avoid nuts that have been roasted or salted, as well as nut butters that have added sweeteners.

dried fruits

Dried cherries

Dried coconut

Dried cranberries

Goji berries

Medjool dates

Raisins

Note: Make sure dried fruit is unsulfured and unsweetened.

sweeteners

Honey

Monk fruit

Pure maple syrup

Stevia

herbs, spices, & extracts

Bay leaves	Himalayan pink salt
Cayenne pepper	Oregano
Chili powder	Paprika
Chipotle powder	Pepper
Cinnamon	Rosemary
Cloves	Smoked paprika
Coriander	Turmeric
Cumin	Almond extract
Curry powder	Vanilla extract
Gomasio	

Note: We've found that using fresh herbs whenever possible makes the world of difference in a recipe.

nongluten grains & pseudograins

Brown rice	Quinoa
Millet	Wild rice
Oats (make sure they are certified gluten-free and organic)	

beans & legumes

Black beans	Lentils (red and green)
Chickpeas (garbanzo beans)	

superfoods

Cacao nibs	Nori sheets
Carob powder	Raw cacao powder
Dulse	Sea vegetables
Maca powder	Spirulina

flours

Almond flour	Oat flour
Arrowroot powder	Rice flour and brown rice flour
Cashew flour	Tiger nut flour
Cassava flour	
Chickpea flour	

other foods

Anchovies	Dairy-free chocolate chips
Artichoke hearts	Dijon mustard
Canned coconut milk	Fish sauce
Chickpea miso	Olives

GO ORGANIC

It's never been more important to source high-quality organic foods than it is today. With poor air quality, EMFs, and unseen chemicals in our food and water, it's critical to reduce our exposure to the toxins found in nonorganic food as much as possible. Take it slowly to adjust to the increased cost of your food bill when buying organics. But remember, you're going to pay the farmer now or pay the doctor later. The money spent today on healthy, organic, whole foods will pay back huge dividends down the road.

---

how to use this book

Whether you're embarking on the 14-day Conscious Cleanse or simply want to eat cleaner, healthier food, it's our hope that the recipes in this book will ignite your senses, tune up your taste buds, and maybe even help you wow a few guests. You don't have to be on the Conscious Cleanse or adopt the 80:20 Plan. If you simply use this cookbook as the mood strikes, you will increase your energy and overall well-being.

Use the recipes in this cookbook as a gateway to explore how food makes you feel. Experiment, have fun, and try new foods. As you do, you'll naturally be diving deeper into the concepts of clean eating, cleansing, optimizing digestion, healing the gut, reducing inflammation, and identifying food sensitivities.

The recipes in this cookbook are best when shared. Invite friends over. Cook for your family. Enjoy eating new foods together. Include your kids in meal planning and preparation. Get your hands dirty and know that you cannot fail here. Simply get into the kitchen, and be curious and adventurous. Your new—vibrant— normal starts now!

TAKE IT ONE STEP AT A TIME

Over the years of teaching ourselves how to cook and become more proficient in the kitchen, we've realized there is great power in learning to master a few recipes. So, find three to five recipes in this book that speak to you and make them over and over again, until you can make them by heart. Pick one smoothie, a salad dressing, a soup, a meat or seafood dish, and a dessert. Have fun mastering them. As you do this, your confidence will soar, increasing your willingness to play even more in the kitchen. Before you know it, you'll be whipping up your own variations and creations. Be gentle with yourself as you start your journey in the kitchen. Blunders and mishaps are part of the exploratory process.

EAT WHAT YOU LIKE

There are many misconceptions when it comes to cleansing. We once had a cleanse participant tell us she "hated kale" and therefore assumed she was "doomed for cleanse failure." This couldn't be further from the truth. Part of becoming food conscious is being willing to try new things—as you clean up your diet, your taste buds might change, so be excited about that! However, if you don't like kale, don't eat kale. If you wake up one day and don't feel like eating chicken anymore, by all means, stop eating chicken. Your body has innate wisdom, and part of the cleansing process is clearing away all the muck and mire so you can tune in to this wise, intuitive part of yourself.

BE FLEXIBLE

As yoga teachers, we know that being flexible has very little to do with being able to touch your toes. It does, however, require practice and patience. Whether you're on your yoga mat or in the kitchen, flexibility is a mindset. Learning to be flexible with the recipes and ingredients takes practice. It also means that you might not create the perfect masterpiece every time, and that's okay. If you find that you've forgotten an ingredient at the store, improvise! If you're inspired to alter the recipe, do that, too! Go with your gut, trust your inner knowing, and above all else, have fun. Being in the kitchen should be joyful. Remember, energy is everything. So be mindful of what you're infusing your food with!

RECIPE ICONS EXPLAINED

To help you quickly navigate the recipes, we've created the following icons. At a glance, you'll know if the recipes fits your needs, whether you're on the cleanse, living the 80:20, or watching your sugar.

CLEANSE = CONSCIOUS CLEANSE APPROVED

These recipes are Conscious Cleanse friendly and perfect for the 14-day cleanse and beyond. Our hope is that you find this so-called "cleanse food" to be so delicious that it becomes part of your regular rotation on and off the cleanse.

80:20 = 80:20 FRIENDLY

These recipes are for living the 80:20 lifestyle. While all of these recipes are major upgrades in terms of offering greater nutrient density and low-sugar alternatives, they fall into the 80:20 category for two main reasons. Either the recipe contains ingredients that are not on the Conscious Cleanse, or it does not follow easy-in, easy-out food combining guidelines. In the case of food combining, look at the recipe notes for simple modifications to make the recipe cleanse-friendly.

LS = LOW SUGAR

Low-sugar recipes contain no more than 1 cup of low-glycemic fruit and do not contain any grains, beans, dried fruit, or natural sweeteners like maple syrup or honey.

Everything in this cookbook is dairy-free, gluten-free, soy-free, and peanut-free.

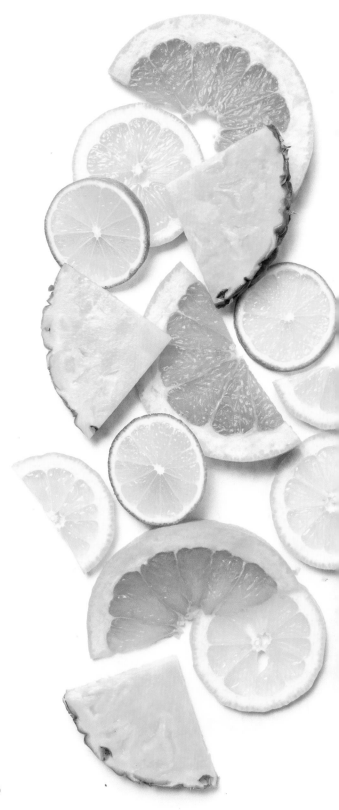

smoothies & juices

natural bzzz green smoothie 43

jo's super green smoothie.. 44

cran-pear smoothie 46

green ollie smoothie 46

carrot cake in a bowl 47

apple pie smoothie 47

"get the glow" green smoothie................................ 48

mint chocolate chip smoothie 48

the great eliminator 49

spirulina smoothie 49

dragon fruit smoothie bowl 51

real-deal protein powders...................................... 52

mint green sweetie smoothie.................................. 53

chocolate cherry smoothie 53

lemon blueberry smoothie...................................... 54

power-up protein smoothie 56

lemon lime cucumber cooler................................... 57

heavy metals be gone juice 58

cardio booster juice 58

jules' go-to green juice 59

spicy greens juice 59

immune blaster juice shot...................................... 61

how to build a green smoothie

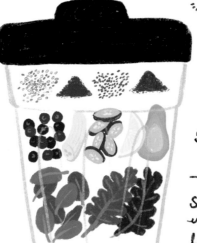

blend until smooth & creamy!

STEP 4: Add a *boost!*

STEP 3: choose some fruit

STEP 2: Load up on dark leafy greens

STEP 1: start with 2 cups of base liquid

Green smoothies have long been our number-one secret to vibrant health! Select a base, like water, nut milk, or coconut water. Fill the blender with dark leafy greens, like spinach or kale. Throw in a cup or two of fruit for sweetness (optional), and finally, pick a superfood boost, like chia seeds, flaxseeds, or spirulina. Blend until smooth, and there you have it—nature's perfect fast food!

natural bzzz green smoothie

Looking for a protein-packed green smoothie that will give you energy to last all morning? Look no further! Tahini and hemp seeds deliver essential amino acids and protein, and a scoop of tiny-but-mighty bee pollen boosts nutrient absorption and balances hormones.

	Yield **1 quart**	Prep Time **5 minutes**	Cook Time **None**	CLEANSE

2 cups water

2 cups frozen mango

2 cups spinach, packed

1 tbsp raw tahini (Artisana Organics brand recommended)

2 tbsp hemp seeds

1 tbsp bee pollen (see note)

½ tsp pure vanilla extract

In a high-speed blender, combine all ingredients. Blend until smooth and creamy. Enjoy immediately.

note

Packed with complex B vitamins, antioxidants, amino acids, and protein, bee pollen is a nutritional powerhouse. Good for allergies, inflammation, energy, and immunity, there isn't much these golden granules can't do. Most health food stores carry bee pollen as a supplement, but when possible, source it from your local beekeeper.

jo's super green smoothie

If you want something simple and earthy that will power you up, you'll love this nutrient-dense green wonder. The best part? It's all veggie, no fruit—perfect for those on the Low Sugar Track.

Yield **1 quart**	Prep Time **5 minutes**	Cook Time **None**	CLEANSE

2 cups water

1 heaping handful of spinach

½ cucumber, cut into chunks

Juice of ½ lemon

2 stalks celery, cut into chunks

½ cup (or ½ handful) fresh cilantro

½ cup (or ½ handful) fresh Italian (flat-leaf) parsley

1–2-in piece fresh ginger, peeled and cut into chunks

In a high-speed blender, combine all ingredients. Blend until smooth. Enjoy immediately!

tip

If you prefer a colder smoothie, replace ½ cup water with ½ cup crushed ice.

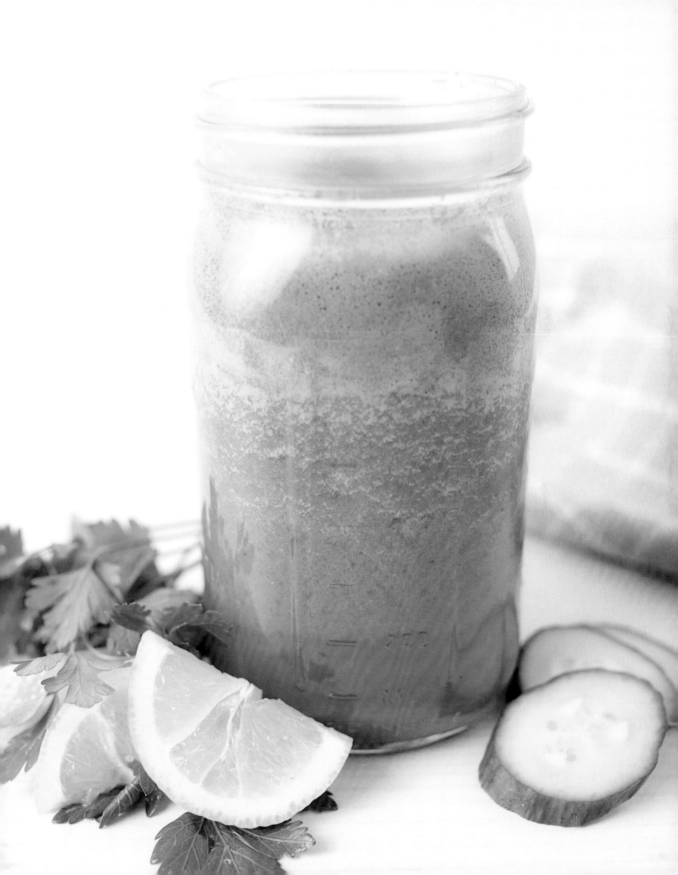

cran-pear smoothie

This is one of Jo's favorite low-sugar smoothies featuring two low-glycemic fruits: cranberries and pear. Cranberries are considered a superfood due to their high nutrient and antioxidant content.

Yield **1 quart**	Prep Time **5 minutes, plus overnight soak**	Cook Time **None**	CLEANSE

2 cups water

1 heaping handful of spinach

¼ cup frozen cranberries

1 large ripe pear, cut into chunks

¼ cup raw cashews, soaked overnight and drained

1 tsp ground cinnamon

In a high-speed blender, combine all ingredients. Blend for about 1 minute to get a smooth and creamy consistency. Enjoy immediately!

tip
You can give the cashews a quick soak for 1 hour to soften them, but it's preferable to soak them overnight for maximum absorption and creaminess.

green ollie smoothie

Olive oil in a green smoothie? Yes, please! Refreshing and satiating, this low-sugar green smoothie will fight inflammation while giving your heart and brain more support. Use a high-quality, organic, extra-virgin olive oil to maximize the benefits of this amazing superfood.

Yield **1 quart**	Prep Time **5 minutes**	Cook Time **None**	CLEANSE

1½ cups water

Juice of ½ lemon

1½-in piece fresh ginger, peeled and cut into chunks

3 romaine lettuce leaves

½ cucumber, cut into chunks

1 cup baby spinach

1 ripe pear, cut into chunks

1 tbsp olive oil

Handful of ice (optional)

In a high-speed blender, combine all ingredients. Blend until smooth and creamy. Enjoy!

carrot cake in a bowl

We love transforming our favorite desserts into nutrient-dense bundles of health-promoting goodness. Packed with beta-carotene and spice, this carrot cake smoothie is everything nice … in a bowl! Top with your favorite add-ons, like our Grain-Free Nutty Granola, pecans, or shredded coconut.

Yield **1–2 servings**	Prep Time **5 minutes**	Cook Time **None**	CLEANSE

1 cup **Coconut Milk** (page 231)

1 banana, frozen

1 cup chopped carrot

¼ avocado

1-in piece fresh ginger, peeled and cut into chunks

1 cup spinach or romaine lettuce

1 tsp ground cinnamon

⅛ tsp ground nutmeg

½ tsp pure vanilla extract

In a high-speed blender, combine all ingredients. Blend until smooth. Pour into bowls, and enjoy immediately!

apple pie smoothie

This smoothie gives you all the flavors of apple pie without the sugar crash. One of our favorite low-sugar smoothies, this recipe features apples, which are low on the glycemic index, a great source of fiber, and rich in immune-boosting vitamin C. Plus, cinnamon helps to regulate blood sugar levels.

Yield **3 cups**	Prep Time **5 minutes**	Cook Time **None**	LS CLEANSE

2 cups **Almond Milk** (page 230)

1 apple, cut into chunks (green if you like it tart, red if you like it sweet)

2 cups spinach

1-in piece fresh ginger, peeled and cut into chunks

1 tsp ground cinnamon

¼ tsp ground nutmeg

Handful of ice (optional)

In a high-speed blender, combine all ingredients. Blend until smooth. Enjoy!

variation

For a warm smoothie, run the blender a little longer than usual (1–2 minutes will do the trick) until the drinking temperature is to your liking.

"get the glow" green smoothie

Want to know the truth about youthful, radiant-looking skin? It comes from the inside! Packed with vitamins, minerals, and healthy fats, this potent beauty elixir delivers. It also helps to detox and hydrate, two more essentials to glowing skin.

Yield **1 quart**	Prep Time **5 minutes**	Cook Time **None**	CLEANSE

1½ cups plain coconut water

1 large cucumber, cut into chunks

2 heaping handfuls of baby kale

Juice of 1 lemon

½ avocado, frozen

1 ripe pear, cut into chunks
  (or stevia, to taste)

In a high-speed blender, combine all ingredients. Blend until creamy, and enjoy immediately.

note

Pasteurized boxed coconut water is not ideal and tends to be high in sugar. If you can find fresh young coconut, that's the best choice. However, when convenience wins out, we reach for Harmless Harvest organic coconut water.

mint chocolate chip smoothie

Better than mint chocolate chip ice cream, this magical concoction has all the healthy magnificence of the refreshing flavor combination we love, without the bloat or sugar rush.

Yield **1 quart**	Prep Time **5 minutes**	Cook Time **None**	80:20

1 (13.5oz) can full-fat coconut milk, chilled for at least 4 hours

½ cup plain coconut water

1½ cups spinach

¼ cup fresh mint leaves

2 bananas, frozen

1 tsp coconut oil

¼ tsp peppermint extract

5–10 drops of liquid stevia (optional)

2 tbsp cacao nibs

1 In a high-speed blender, combine the coconut milk, coconut water, spinach, mint, bananas, coconut oil, peppermint, and stevia, if using. Blend on high until smooth.

2 Set the blender to low, add the cacao nibs, and blend for 5 seconds. Top with more cacao nibs, and serve immediately.

the great eliminator

As its name suggests, this smoothie is designed to help you get things moving. The trifecta of dandelion greens (a diuretic and great source of prebiotics), sprouts (high in living enzymes and good for digestion), and flaxseeds (a well-known remedy for constipation) do the trick to move the gunk out.

Yield **1 quart**	Prep Time **5 minutes**	Cook Time **None**	CLEANSE

2 cups water

1 cup spinach

½ bunch dandelion greens

½ cup sprouts (any variety)

2 cups frozen peaches

2 tbsp ground flaxseeds

1–2 Medjool dates, pitted, or stevia, to taste

In a high-speed blender, combine all ingredients. Blend until smooth. Enjoy immediately.

spirulina smoothie

Spirulina, along with its cousin, chlorella, is one of the most nutrient-dense foods on the planet. This blue-green algae is our go-to green powder because it's a complete protein that's highly bioavailable.

Yield **1 quart**	Prep Time **5 minutes**	Cook Time **None**	CLEANSE

1 cup **Coconut Milk** (page 231)

1 cup water

1 banana, frozen

1 cup frozen mango

1-in piece fresh ginger, peeled

2 cups spinach

1 tsp spirulina

In a high-speed blender, combine all ingredients. Blend on high until smooth and creamy. Enjoy!

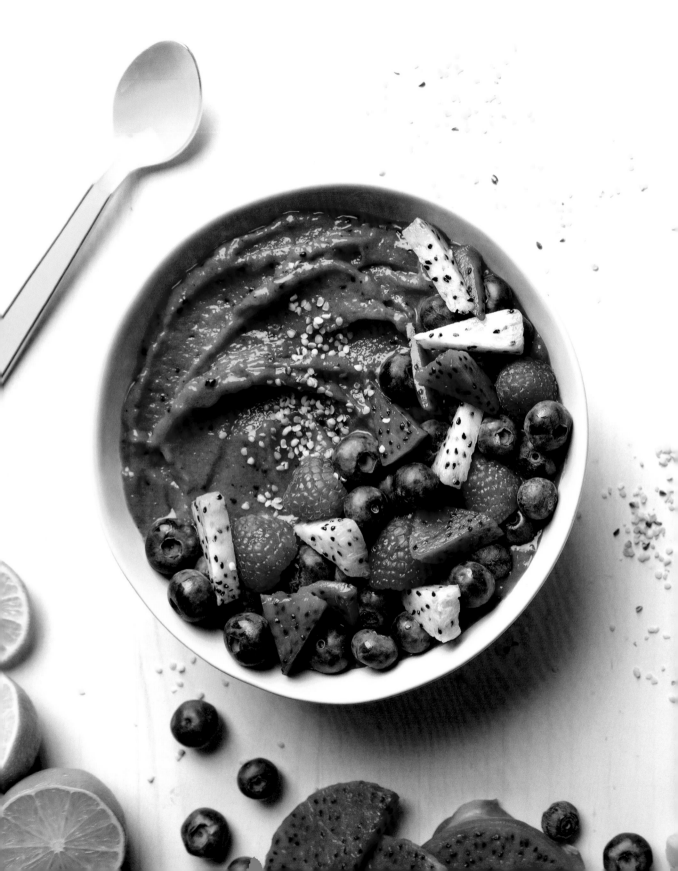

dragon fruit smoothie bowl

Jules' older boys ask for this refreshing smoothie bowl by name! Dragon fruit, also called pitaya, is a superfood known for rejuvenating the liver and delivering a hefty dose of antioxidants. It brings a vivid pink color and sweetness to this bowl—your kids might think you're letting them eat sorbet for breakfast!

Yield **2 servings**	Prep Time **15 minutes**	Cook Time **None**	CLEANSE

2 (100g) dragon fruit (pitaya) smoothie packs (Pitaya Plus brand recommended)

1 cup frozen mango

½ avocado, frozen

1 banana, frozen

1-in piece fresh ginger, peeled and cut into chunks

Juice of ½ lime

Handful of romaine lettuce

To garnish (optional)
Fresh dragon fruit, fresh berries, granola, shredded coconut

1 In a high-speed blender, combine all ingredients. Blend on low until smooth and creamy, using the tamper if needed to push down the ingredients. (Keeping the setting on low is the key to a smooth, creamy consistency.)

2 Transfer to a bowl, and top with desired garnishes.

tip
To keep cleanse friendly, only garnish with fresh fruit (not granola).

real-deal protein powders

One of the most frequent questions we get is, "Can I use protein powder while on the cleanse?" We always prefer "the real deal," so we made our own less-processed, plant-based versions using hemp and chia seeds. Choose from three flavorful variations to give your smoothie or homemade nut milk a protein boost.

Yield **2 cups**	Prep Time **5 minutes**	Cook Time **None**	LS CLEANSE

Cinnamon Spice Hemp

2 cups hemp seeds

2 tbsp ground cinnamon

1 tsp ground nutmeg

2 tbsp Lakanto Classic Monkfruit
  Sweetener (optional)

Chia Cinnamon with a Kick

2 cups chia seeds

2–3 tbsp ground cinnamon

1–2 tsp cayenne pepper

2 tbsp cacao powder

2 tbsp Lakanto Classic Monkfruit
  Sweetener

Chocolate Hemp (80:20)

2 cups hemp seeds

2 tbsp raw cacao powder

2 tbsp Lakanto Classic Monkfruit
  Sweetener (optional)

1 In a food processor, combine all ingredients for your flavor blend of choice. Process until the mixture reaches a powder-like consistency, but take care not to overblend. (The mixture will not be a fine powder like a commercial protein powder, but a bit chunkier.) Transfer to an airtight container, and refrigerate to preserve freshness.

2 To use, mix 3 tablespoons protein powder with 2 cups homemade nut milk or blend into your favorite smoothie.

mint green sweetie smoothie

Fresh mint is a secret superfood. Refreshing, naturally sweet, and low in sugar, this is one of our new favorite go-tos. The addition of fresh herbs, like mint, automatically gives smoothies more flavor and nutrients. We use our homemade protein powder here, which is packed with protein from hemp seeds.

Yield **3 cups**	Prep Time **5 minutes**	Cook Time **None**	CLEANSE

2 cups water

2 tbsp macadamia nuts

1 tbsp **Cinnamon Spice Hemp Protein Powder** (page 52)

1 cucumber, cut into chunks

3–4 sprigs fresh mint

2–3 handfuls of spinach

8–10 drops of liquid stevia (optional)

In a high-speed blender, combine all ingredients. Blend until smooth. Enjoy!

chocolate cherry smoothie

One of Jules' favorite 80:20 smoothies, this classic combo of chocolate and cherries is perfect after a workout or when you need an extra pick-me-up. Packed with healthy fats and omega-3s, this filling green smoothie will keep you going strong for hours.

Yield **1 quart**	Prep Time **5 minutes**	Cook Time **None**	80:20

2 cups **Almond Milk** (page 230)

1 ripe banana

1 cup frozen cherries

¼ avocado

2 cups spinach or kale

1 tbsp **Chocolate Hemp Protein Powder** (page 52)

1–3 drops of liquid stevia (optional)

In a high-speed blender, combine all ingredients. Blend until smooth. Enjoy!

lemon blueberry smoothie

This is one of our signature low-sugar smoothies that actually tastes a bit like blueberry pie! Bright and zesty, this smoothie features romaine lettuce, which, contrary to popular belief, is a nutrient-dense leafy green, filled with antioxidants like vitamins A and C.

Yield **1 quart**	Prep Time **20 minutes**	Cook Time **None**	**LS** CLEANSE

2 cups **Cashew Milk** (page 230)

1 tbsp chia seeds

3 large romaine lettuce leaves

1 cup spinach

Small handful of fresh Italian (flat-leaf) parsley

¼ tsp lemon zest

Juice of ½ lemon

2 cups frozen blueberries

In a high-speed blender, combine all ingredients. Blend until smooth. Enjoy!

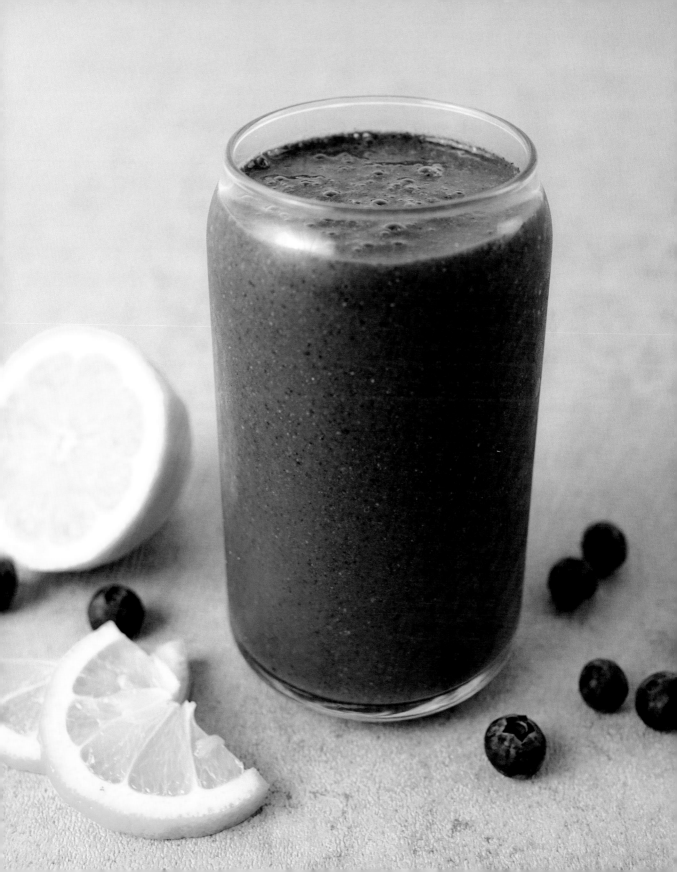

power-up protein smoothie

If you're looking for the perfect post-workout green smoothie, this is it! It's loaded with plant-powered protein and blood sugar–stabilizing superfoods.

Yield **1 quart**	Prep Time **5 minutes**	Cook Time **None**	**LS** CLEANSE

½ cup water

½ cup unsweetened hemp or almond milk

⅔ cup blueberries

⅓ cup cranberries, frozen or fresh

2 handfuls of spinach

1 tsp maca powder

1 tsp ground cinnamon

3 tbsp **Cinnamon Spice Hemp Protein Powder** (page 52)

1 tbsp raw walnut or almond butter

1 tbsp pumpkin seeds

1 tsp chia seeds

In a high-speed blender, combine all ingredients. Blend for 1 minute to get a smooth and creamy consistency. Enjoy immediately!

lemon lime cucumber cooler

Cucumbers are one of nature's best beauty foods. They're full of minerals (especially silica) that promote healthy skin, hair, and nails. Both detoxifying and hydrating, this vivid green juice will delight your taste buds with its burst of citrus twist!

Yield **1 quart**	Prep Time **5 minutes**	Cook Time **None**	**LS** CLEANSE

1 lemon, peeled
1 lime, peeled
1 large cucumber
1 head celery
1 bunch collard greens

In a juicer, combine all ingredients. Pour over ice in a quart-size Mason jar, and enjoy immediately.

heavy metals be gone juice

This powerhouse juice is good preventive medicine. Not for the uninitiated, this super green juice will chelate toxic heavy metals and help to detox the liver and the kidneys.

Yield **1 quart**	Prep Time **10 minutes**	Cook Time **None**	LS CLEANSE

2 lemons, peeled

1 bunch spinach

½ bunch dandelion greens

1 cucumber

1 head celery

1 bunch fresh cilantro

1 bunch fresh Italian (flat-leaf) parsley

In a juicer, combine all ingredients. Pour into a Mason jar, and enjoy immediately.

cardio booster juice

Beets are good for building the blood, which is amazing for boosting cardiovascular health and supercharging a workout! And if liver detox is what you're looking for, beet juice is the answer.

Yield **2½ cups**	Prep Time **10 minutes**	Cook Time **None**	LS CLEANSE

2 medium beets, trimmed and scrubbed

1 large bunch celery

1 large bunch spinach

1 green apple

1 lemon, peeled

In a juicer, combine all ingredients. Pour into a Mason jar, and enjoy immediately.

jules' go-to green juice

This green juice is the non-negotiable foundation of Jules' wellness plan. Hydrating and alkalizing, it's loaded with enzymes and easily absorbed. It's like high-speed nutrition delivered right to your cells.

Yield **1 quart**	Prep Time **5 minutes**	Cook Time **None**	CLEANSE

½ cucumber

6 large kale leaves, with stems

4 collard leaves

½ bunch fresh Italian (flat-leaf) parsley

1 head romaine lettuce

1 head celery

In a juicer, combine all ingredients. Pour into a Mason jar, and enjoy immediately.

spicy greens juice

Looking for a little kick from your green juice? This juice utilizes the stalks from the broccoli bunch that many would toss in the compost. It's clean and simple, delivering hydration, minerals, and vitamins while also boosting digestion.

Yield **1 quart**	Prep Time **5 minutes**	Cook Time **None**	CLEANSE

2 small lemons, peeled

1 head celery

1 cucumber

2 stalks broccoli

½ bunch kale

½ bunch fresh Italian (flat-leaf) parsley

2–2½-in piece fresh ginger

In a juicer, combine all ingredients. Pour into a Mason jar, and enjoy immediately.

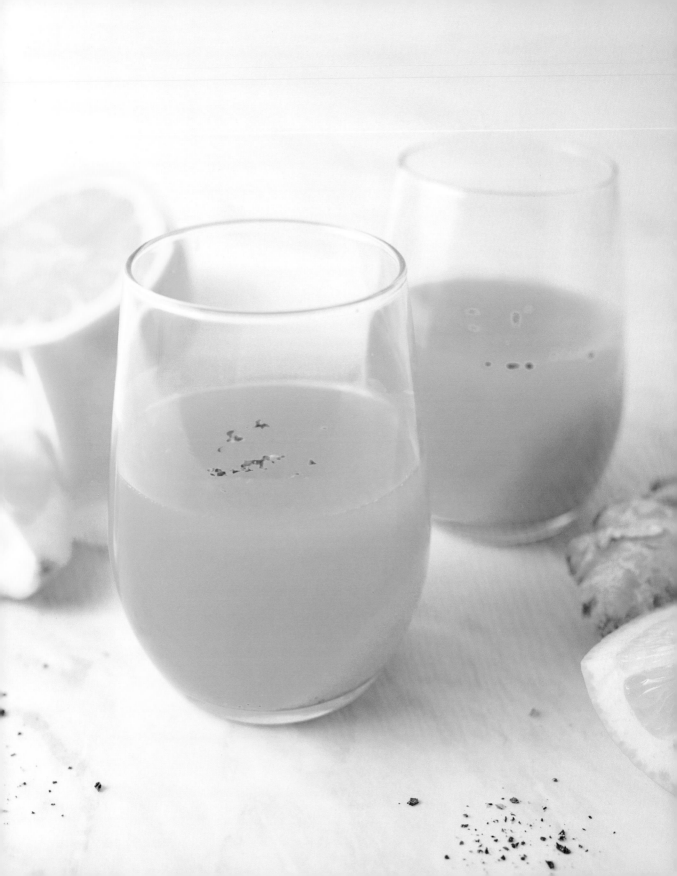

immune blaster juice shot

Feeling under the weather or just want to fortify your immune system? Try knocking back this shot for a blast of vitamin C and anti-inflammatory goodness. Top with a pinch of cayenne pepper for an extra kick!

Yield **2 servings**	Prep Time **10 minutes**	Cook Time **None**	CLEANSE

4-in piece fresh turmeric

4-in piece fresh ginger

4 lemons, peeled

1 tbsp local honey

Freshly ground black pepper

In a juicer, combine turmeric, ginger, and lemons. After juicing, stir in the honey and a few grinds of pepper. Sip immediately.

breakfasts

egg-free veggie scramble 64

baked oatmeal cups 66

five-ingredient breakfast cookies 67

blueberry hemp bites 69

grain-free nutty granola 70

veggie egg muffins 71

dairy-free coconut yogurt 72

breakfast niçoise salad... 74

sardines for breakfast 75

turkey breakfast skillet 77

maple sage breakfast sausage.............................. 78

squashie pancakes 79

egg-free veggie scramble

If you love a warm and veggie-filled breakfast, look no further. Perfect while cleansing, this egg-free scramble can be enjoyed in the morning or any time of the day.

Yield **2 servings**	Prep Time **15 minutes**	Cook Time **10 minutes**	CLEANSE

1 tbsp olive oil

½ shallot, chopped

1 clove garlic, minced

2 cups chopped broccoli

1 cup diced zucchini

½ cup sliced cremini mushrooms

Himalayan pink salt and freshly
  ground black pepper, to taste

1 bunch kale, stems removed,
  chopped

1 avocado, sliced

¼ cup store-bought kimchi

Lemon wedge (optional), to serve

1 In a large sauté pan, heat the oil over medium heat. Add the shallot, and cook for 1 minute. When the shallot is translucent, add the garlic, broccoli, zucchini, mushrooms, and a pinch of salt. Sauté for 2 to 3 minutes.

2 Add the kale, cover, and steam for 2 minutes. Remove the lid, and sauté for 1 minute more until the vegetables are soft.

3 Transfer to plates and top each serving with sliced avocado and kimchi. Season with salt and pepper to taste and a squeeze of lemon, if desired.

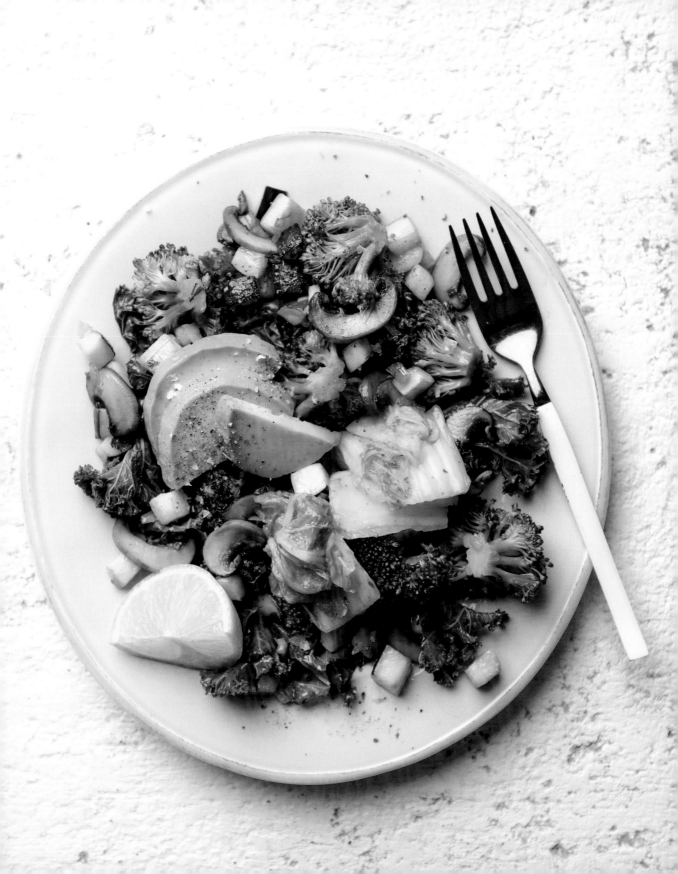

baked oatmeal cups

If you've never had baked oatmeal cups, get ready to have your mind blown. A quick, easy, and portable breakfast or snack, these tender oatmeal cups can be adapted to suit all your eaters. Try one of our suggested add-in options, or come up with flavor combinations of your own. The sky's the limit!

Yield **12 muffins**	Prep Time **10 minutes**	Cook Time **25 minutes**	80:20

2 eggs

1½ cups unsweetened nut milk

½ cup unsweetened applesauce

¼ cup almond butter

¼ cup maple syrup (or Lakanto Classic Monkfruit Sweetener)

1 tsp pure vanilla extract

3 cups gluten-free oats

1 tsp baking powder

1 tsp ground cinnamon

½ tsp Himalayan pink salt

1 cup add-ins (see options)

Add-in options

Dark chocolate chips and dried cherries

Chopped raw walnuts and shredded carrots

Pumpkin seeds and raisins

Shredded zucchini and chopped strawberries

1 Preheat the oven to 350°F, and grease a 12-cup muffin pan.

2 In a large bowl, combine the eggs, nut milk, applesauce, almond butter, maple syrup, and vanilla. Mix until smooth. Add the oats, baking powder, cinnamon, and salt. Stir until well combined.

3 Using a spatula, fold in your favorite add-ins. Divide batter evenly among the muffin cups. Bake for 25 minutes or until golden brown.

4 Cool in the pan for at least 5 minutes before removing. Use a butter knife to loosen each muffin and transfer to a wire rack to cool completely. Store in the refrigerator for up to 1 week.

tip

Oatmeal cups can be individually wrapped and frozen for up to 1 month. Defrost overnight in the refrigerator.

five-ingredient breakfast cookies

Jules and her boys have been making these healthy "cookies" for years. What kid doesn't love a cookie for breakfast? Our go-to recipe when we have overripe bananas, this is sure to become a family favorite!

Yield **24 cookies**	Prep Time **5 minutes**	Cook Time **12 minutes**	80:20

4 ripe bananas, peeled and broken into chunks

2 cups gluten-free oats (see note)

½ cup raisins

1 tsp ground cinnamon

½ tsp Himalayan pink salt

½ cup dairy-free mini chocolate chips (optional)

1   Preheat the oven to 350°F. Line a baking sheet with parchment paper or a silicone liner.

2   In a medium bowl, mash the bananas with a fork until there are no chunks left. Stir in the oats, raisins, cinnamon, salt, and chocolate chips, if using.

3   Using a spoon or cookie scoop, scoop the batter onto the prepared baking sheet. Bake for 12 minutes. Remove from the oven and let cool for 5 minutes then transfer to a wire rack to cool completely. Store in an airtight container for up to 1 week.

note

Make sure to source organic, gluten-free oats. Although gluten-free by nature, oats are often cross-contaminated. Conventionally grown oats have been shown to contain a hefty dose of glyphosate, the weed-killing poison found in Roundup, when tested by the Environmental Working Group.

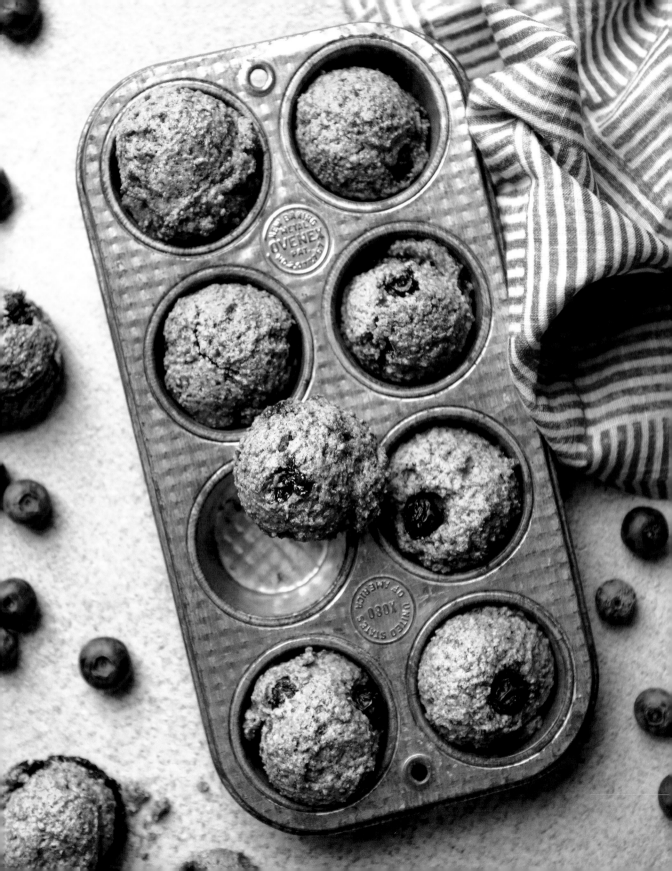

blueberry hemp bites

The perfect blueberry muffin: gluten-free (of course!), vegan, and grain-free. Thanks to the hemp seeds, these make a delicious, protein-packed, grab-and-go breakfast both you and your kids will devour.

Yield **12 bites**	Prep Time **10 minutes**	Cook Time **30 minutes**	LS 80:20

1 tbsp ground flaxseeds

3 tbsp water

1½ cups hemp seeds

¼ cup cassava flour (see note)

¼ tsp Himalayan pink salt

1 tsp ground cinnamon

3 tbsp Lakanto Classic Monkfruit Sweetener

1 tsp pure vanilla extract

¼ cup unsweetened nut milk

½ cup fresh blueberries

1 Preheat the oven to 350°F. Grease a 12-cup muffin pan with olive or coconut oil or use silicone liners. In a small bowl, whisk together the ground flaxseeds and water. Set aside to thicken for 10 minutes.

2 In a food processor, blend the hemp seeds to a fine powder. Add the cassava flour, salt, cinnamon, and sweetener. Pulse gently to mix ingredients. Transfer the mixture to a medium bowl.

3 Add the vanilla and nut milk to the bowl with the flaxseeds, and whisk to combine. Add the flaxseed mixture to the hemp seed mixture, and mix thoroughly. Fold in the blueberries. Spoon a heaping tablespoon of batter into each muffin cup. Bake for 25 to 30 minutes.

4 Remove from the oven and let the hemp bites cool completely before eating. Store in an airtight container in the refrigerator for up to 5 days.

note

Cassava flour is gluten-, grain-, and nut-free. It's high in resistant starch, which is great for helping to regulate blood sugar.

grain-free nutty granola

If you're looking for a power-packed breakfast that will keep you feeling full, this granola is for you. High in healthy fats and omega-3s and free of grains, it is delicious with nut milk or as a quick snack.

Yield **8 servings**	Prep Time **10 minutes**	Cook Time **15 minutes**	CLEANSE

1 cup raw pecans

1 cup raw cashews

¼ cup raw pumpkin seeds

¼ cup raw sunflower seeds

¼ cup whole flaxseeds

¼ cup ground flaxseeds

3 tbsp chia seeds

2 tbsp olive oil

2 tbsp maple syrup (or Lakanto Classic Monkfruit Sweetener for low sugar)

1 tsp pure vanilla extract

2 tsp ground cinnamon

1 tsp Himalayan pink salt

1 Preheat the oven to 350°F. Line a baking sheet with parchment paper.

2 In a food processor, pulse the pecans, cashews, pumpkin seeds, sunflower seeds, whole and ground flaxseeds, and chia seeds 3 to 4 times to break into small chunks. (Take care not to overblend, or your mixture will be too fine.)

3 In a large bowl, whisk together the olive oil, maple syrup, vanilla, cinnamon, and salt. Slowly incorporate the ground nut mixture into the bowl, and stir until everything is fully coated.

4 Spread the granola mixture evenly onto the prepared baking sheet, and bake for 12 to 15 minutes or until lightly browned. Stir once halfway through baking. Remove from the oven and let cool completely before transferring to an airtight glass container for storage.

veggie egg muffins

These are perfect for an on-the-go breakfast and are so easy to customize. Have fun experimenting and finding your favorite "fillings." We like to pack in as many veggies and dark leafy greens as possible.

Yield **12 muffins**	Prep Time **15 minutes**	Cook Time **20 minutes**	80:20

8 eggs

¼ cup plain, unsweetened coconut milk

¾ tsp Himalayan pink salt

¼ tsp freshly ground black pepper

3 tbsp nutritional yeast

1 cup spinach, packed, cut into ribbons

¼ cup sun-dried tomatoes, soaked for 1 hour, drained, and chopped

¼ cup finely chopped red onion

1 Preheat the oven to 350°F. Line a 12-cup muffin pan with silicone liners.

2 In a large bowl, whisk the eggs with the coconut milk, salt, pepper, and nutritional yeast.

3 In a separate bowl, combine the spinach, tomatoes, and red onion. Divide the vegetable mixture among the 12 muffin cups and then pour the egg mixture over top, filling the cups about two-thirds full.

4 Bake for 20 minutes or until the centers are set. Test by inserting a toothpick into the center of a muffin. They are done if the toothpick comes out clean.

5 Remove from the oven and let the muffins cool in the pan for at least 20 minutes. Transfer to a cooling rack, or serve warm. Refrigerate muffins in an airtight container for up to 3 days. To reheat, preheat the oven to 400°F. Place muffins on a baking sheet, and warm for 5 to 7 minutes.

variation

Looking for other delicious filling combinations? Try Swiss chard, shredded sweet potato, and shallot. We also love mushrooms, cherry tomatoes, and zucchini.

dairy-free coconut yogurt
WITH CHIA BERRY JAM

Most store-bought yogurts, whether dairy-free or not, are full of sugar and preservatives. Our coconut variation delivers a cleanse-friendly bowl of creamy yumminess.

Yield **2 servings**	Prep Time **10 minutes**	Cook Time **20 minutes**	CLEANSE

For the jam
1 lb fresh berries, such as raspberries, blackberries, or blueberries

3 tbsp organic honey (adjust to taste depending on sweetness of berries)

½ vanilla bean, split and scraped

2 tbsp chia seeds

Juice of ¼ lemon

For the yogurt
2 (8oz) packets frozen fresh young coconut purée (Inner-Ēco brand recommended), thawed

¼–½ cup coconut water

½ tsp pure vanilla extract

Coconut flakes (optional), to garnish

1 In a medium saucepan, heat the berries, honey, and vanilla bean scrapings over medium-high heat. Bring to a simmer, and cook for 10 minutes or until the juice from the berries has thickened slightly.

2 Add the chia seeds and lemon juice, and continue to cook for 5 to 10 minutes or until the mixture has a jam-like consistency. (It will continue to thicken slightly while cooling.) Transfer to a glass jar, and cool completely before adding to yogurt.

3 In a high-speed blender, combine the coconut purée, ¼ cup coconut water, and vanilla. Blend on high, adding more coconut water if necessary to get the mixture to a consistency similar to Greek yogurt.

4 Serve the yogurt topped with chia berry jam and coconut flakes, if desired. Leftover jam can be refrigerated in an airtight container for up to 7 days.

tip

To boost this yogurt's healing power, stir in the contents of 1 to 2 capsules of your favorite probiotic powder to each serving before eating.

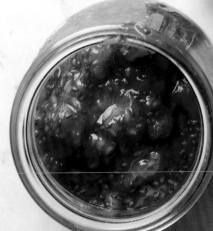

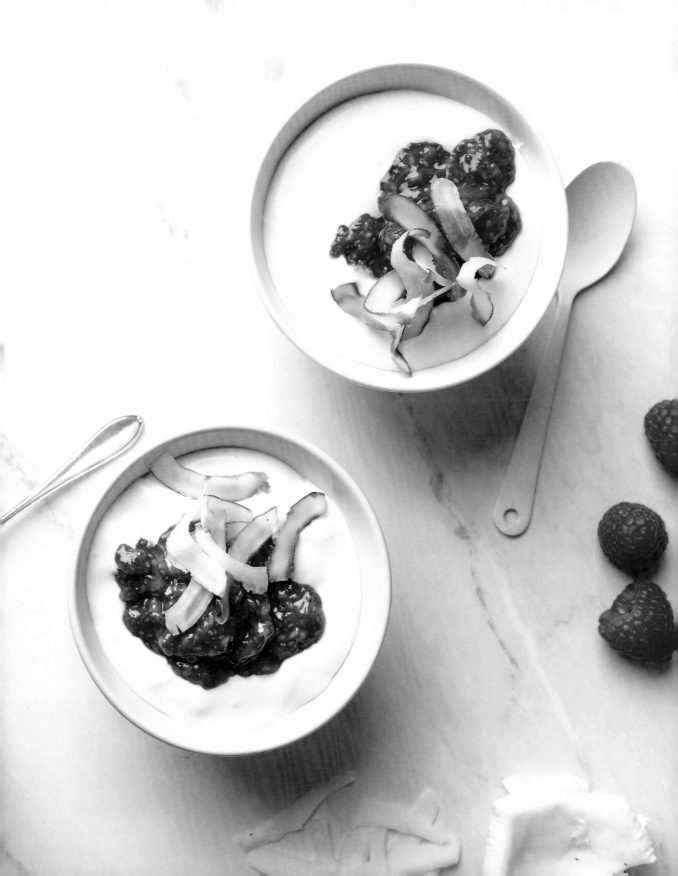

breakfast niçoise salad
WITH LEMON THYME VINAIGRETTE

Salad for breakfast? Why not! Dark leafy greens are one of our staples, especially at breakfast time. So when you're not feeling a green smoothie, have a breakfast salad—and a green smoothie for lunch!

Yield **1 serving**	Prep Time **20 minutes**	Cook Time **10 minutes**	CLEANSE

1 tbsp olive oil

1 bunch radishes, trimmed and halved

1 cup haricots verts (thin French green beans)

2 tbsp sesame seeds

1 tbsp smoked paprika

¼ tsp Himalayan pink salt

¼ lb fresh ahi tuna

1 tbsp coconut oil

2 cups pea shoots or microgreens

3 tbsp sliced green and black olives

For the dressing
Juice of 1 lemon

3 tbsp chopped fresh thyme

1 tsp Dijon mustard

½ clove garlic

Pinch of Himalayan pink salt

Pinch of freshly ground black pepper

3 tbsp olive oil

1 In a small skillet, heat the olive oil over medium heat. Sauté the radishes for about 3 minutes, making sure to keep them slightly crisp. Remove the radishes from the skillet and set aside to cool.

2 In a large saucepan with a steamer insert, steam the green beans over medium-high heat for 5 minutes. Remove from the heat, and run under cold water to keep the green beans bright and crisp. Set aside.

3 On a small plate, combine the sesame seeds, smoked paprika, and salt. Coat the tuna steak with the spice mixture on all four sides. In the same small skillet used to sauté the radishes, heat the coconut oil over medium-high heat. Once hot, sear the tuna on all sides until cooked to your desired doneness (a quick sear on all sides for rare or 5–6 minutes total for medium rare). Let the tuna rest while you make the dressing.

4 To make the dressing, in a high-speed blender, combine the lemon juice, thyme, Dijon mustard, garlic, salt, and pepper. Blend until smooth. Turn blender to low. With the blender running, slowly drizzle in the olive oil.

5 Place the pea shoots in a serving dish. Arrange the radishes, green beans, and olives on top. Thinly slice the tuna steak, and place it over top of the salad. Drizzle with dressing, and enjoy!

tip
Add a hard-boiled or poached egg to the salad if you're not cleansing.

sardines for breakfast

Jo is notorious for busting open a can of sardines for breakfast, so we knew we had to include this recipe in our cookbook. Packed with omega-3s and vitamin B_{12}, this tiny but mighty "super" fish is worth including in your rotation, especially if you're fighting inflammation and want to boost brain health.

Yield **2–4 servings**	Prep Time **10 minutes**	Cook Time **None**	CLEANSE

2 (4.5oz) cans wild sardines (skinless, boneless fillets in olive oil)

½ cup diced red onion

2 tbsp sugar-free relish

1 tsp Dijon mustard

½ avocado, sliced

Freshly ground black pepper, to taste

Mixed greens, arugula, or sautéed chard, to serve

Sliced lemon, to serve

1 In a medium bowl, mash the sardines with a fork. Add the onion, relish, mustard, avocado, and pepper. Stir to combine.

2 Serve on a bed of mixed greens, arugula, or sautéed chard. Top with a squeeze of lemon juice.

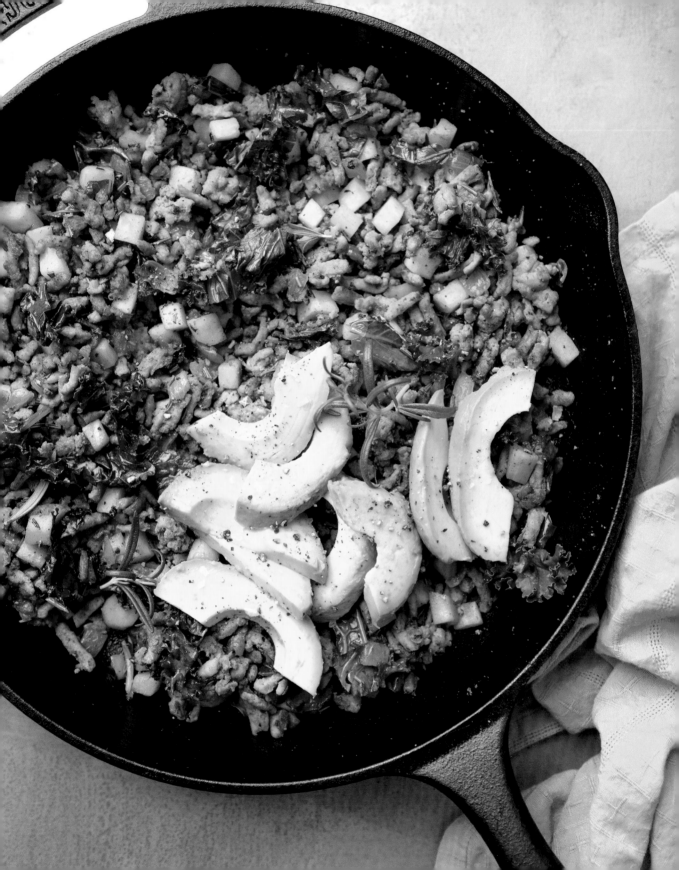

turkey breakfast skillet

This one-pan recipe is a warm and comforting upgrade to the typical bacon-and-egg breakfast, especially during the colder months. Parsnips steal the show with their sweet flavor and potato-like consistency.

Yield **4 servings**	Prep Time **5 minutes**	Cook Time **25 minutes**	CLEANSE

2 tbsp olive oil or coconut oil

1 yellow onion, finely chopped

1 lb ground turkey

1 clove garlic, minced

2 large parsnips, diced

2 tbsp chopped fresh rosemary, divided

1 tsp paprika

½ tsp red pepper flakes

Himalayan pink salt and freshly ground black pepper, to taste

2 cups chopped leafy greens (Swiss chard, kale, spinach, or collard greens)

Sliced avocado (optional), to serve

1 In a sauté pan, heat the oil over medium heat. Add the onion, and cook for 5 minutes or until the onions are soft and translucent.

2 Add the ground turkey, and cook for 5 minutes or until the meat is no longer pink. Add the garlic, and cook for 2 minutes more until the garlic is fragrant and the meat is browned.

3 Add the parsnips, 1 tablespoon rosemary, paprika, and red pepper flakes. Cook for 10 minutes or until the parsnips become tender. Taste and season with salt and pepper.

4 Add the greens, and cook for about 3 minutes or until wilted. Add the remaining 1 tablespoon rosemary, mix well, and serve hot, topped with sliced avocado, if desired.

maple sage breakfast sausage

Breakfast sausage is a staple in our households, but most are filled with sugar or toxic preservatives. This recipe is flavorful but not too spicy, and best of all, it contains a secret superfood—chicken liver! Ounce for ounce, chicken livers are more nutritionally dense than any other food. They're chock-full of vitamin A, iron, and B vitamins like B_{12}. We hope this becomes one of your family favorites, too.

Yield **18 patties**	Prep Time **30 minutes**	Cook Time **40 minutes**	CLEANSE

1 tbsp olive oil

8 oz chicken livers

2 lb ground turkey

1½ tbsp maple syrup

2 tbsp minced fresh sage

2 tsp minced fresh thyme

1 tsp fennel seeds

¼ tsp ground cinnamon

¼ tsp ground nutmeg

1½ tsp Himalayan pink salt

Freshly ground black pepper, to taste

1 Preheat the oven to 350°F. Line a baking sheet with foil.

2 In a medium skillet, heat the oil over medium-high heat. Once hot, add chicken livers, and cook for 4 to 5 minutes on each side, until firm and grayish brown. Transfer to a food processor, and pulse the chicken livers until coarsely ground.

3 In a medium bowl, combine the turkey, maple syrup, sage, thyme, fennel, cinnamon, nutmeg, salt, and pepper. Add the ground chicken livers, and mix well.

4 Using your hands, form heaping tablespoons of the mixture into about 18 patties, and place them on the prepared baking sheet. Bake for 25 to 30 minutes or until the sausage reaches an internal temperature of 165°F.

5 Set the broiler to high, and place a rack 3 inches from the heat source. Brown the sausage patties for 1 minute on each side. Serve warm.

squashie pancakes

Traditional pancakes are flour-based gut-bombs, so Jo and her husband created this recipe for their daughter. Super simple and veggie-centric, this is a tasty alternative that kids and adults alike will love.

Yield **8–10 pancakes**	Prep Time **5 minutes**	Cook Time **1½ hours**	80:20

1 small butternut squash, or
  2 acorn squash

2 tbsp Lakanto Classic Monkfruit
  Sweetener

3 tbsp olive oil, divided

¼ cup water or unsweetened
  nut milk

1 tsp pure vanilla extract

¾ cup cassava flour

½ tsp baking powder

1 Preheat the oven to 400°F. Halve the squash and remove the seeds. Place in a shallow baking dish, cut side up. Add a small amount of water to the dish, enough to fill it about ½ inch. Roast for 60 to 90 minutes or until tender, turning cut side down halfway through baking to caramelize. (Cook time will vary depending on the size of the squash; check for tenderness at 60 minutes.)

2 When the squash is cool enough to handle, scoop the flesh from the skin, and place 2 cups roasted squash in a large bowl. (Any leftover squash can be reserved for another use.) Add to the bowl the sweetener, 2 tablespoons oil, water or nut milk, and vanilla. Mix until well combined.

3 In a separate medium bowl, combine the flour and baking powder; mix thoroughly. Add the dry ingredients to the wet ingredients, and stir to combine.

4 Preheat the oven to 350°F. In a 12-inch oven-safe skillet or griddle, heat the remaining 1 tablespoon oil over medium-low heat. Scoop ⅛-cup portions of the batter into the hot skillet to create pancakes about 4 inches in diameter. Cook for 3 to 4 minutes per side, until browned. Place the skillet in the oven for about 10 minutes to complete cooking. Serve hot.

tip

The roasted squash can be prepared up to 3 days in advance and refrigerated in an airtight container until ready to use.

salads

simple kale salad 83

jules' salad of abundance 84

greek wedge salad 86

spicy kale caesar 87

thai flank steak salad.......................................89

creamy vegan coleslaw....................................90

gut-healing slaw...91

fall harvest salad 92

hemp seed tabbouleh 94

butter lettuce salad 95

mason jar chopped salad 97

warm kale & beet rice salad 98

winter roasted veggie salad 99

thai cucumber noodle salad................................ 100

autumn wild rice salad 102

quinoa watercress salad.......................................103

carrot top pesto salad 105

how to build a salad

STEP 1: choose some leafy greens

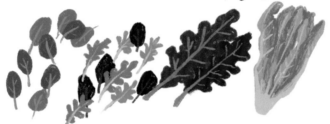

STEP 2: Load up on non-starchy veggies

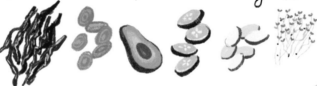

STEP 3: choose an animal protein, starch, nuts, or seeds

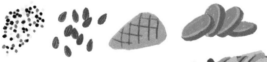

STEP 4: Top with dressing and enjoy!

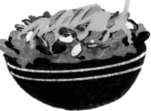

Our big and bountiful "meal-sized" salads begin with a large bowl filled with fresh greens. We then add an array of colorful veggies and sprouts, a plant or animal protein, and a creamy salad dressing.

simple kale salad
WITH HONEY MUSTARD VINAIGRETTE

Who doesn't love a simple massaged kale salad? The trick here is to get your hands dirty (well, wash them first, then dive in) and massage the kale with high-quality olive oil and a generous pinch of Himalayan pink salt. This is one of our regular go-to salads. It's delicious on its own or with our Chipotle Lime Salmon.

Yield **2–4 servings**	Prep Time **15 minutes**	Cook Time **None**	CLEANSE

1 bunch kale, trimmed, stems removed, cut into fine ribbons

½ tbsp olive oil

¼ tsp Himalayan pink salt, or to taste

1 cup shredded red cabbage

1 cup grated carrots

¼ red onion, thinly sliced

2 ripe avocados, chopped

Freshly ground black pepper, to taste

For the dressing

¼ cup olive oil

1½ tsp honey

3 tbsp Dijon mustard

2 tbsp freshly squeezed lemon juice

¼ tsp Himalayan pink salt, or to taste

1 Place the kale in a large salad bowl, and add the olive oil and salt. Using your hands, massage the kale lightly for about 30 seconds. Set aside.

2 To make the dressing, in a small bowl, whisk together all dressing ingredients.

3 Add the cabbage, carrots, onion, and avocados to the kale, and toss to combine. Pour the dressing over the salad, and toss well. Season with pepper to taste.

jules' salad of abundance

The ideal meal-sized salad—overflowing with dark leafy greens and garden-fresh veggies, loaded with sprouts, and drizzled with a hearty dressing—is as filling as it is nutritious. Use this recipe as a guide, and get creative. Have fun and represent a rainbow of colors for maximum nutrient density.

Yield **2 servings**	Prep Time **15 minutes, plus overnight soak**	Cook Time **None**	CLEANSE

4 cups spring greens

1 cup alfalfa sprouts

½ cup sliced radishes

1 cucumber, chopped

½ cup finely shredded red cabbage

1 avocado, sliced

For the dressing

½ cup raw sunflower seeds, soaked overnight and drained

1 clove garlic

1 tbsp lemon zest

¾ cups filtered water

1 tbsp coconut aminos

¾ cup olive oil

2 tbsp freshly squeezed lemon juice

Himalayan pink salt and freshly ground black pepper, to taste

1 To make the dressing, in a high-speed blender, combine the sunflower seeds, garlic, lemon zest, filtered water, coconut aminos, oil, and lemon juice. Blend until smooth. Taste and season with salt and pepper.

2 To assemble the salad, in a large bowl, combine the spring greens, sprouts, radishes, cucumber, cabbage, and avocado. Toss with desired amount of dressing, and serve. Leftover dressing can be refrigerated in an airtight glass jar for up to 1 week.

variation

Toss in your favorite protein! Walnuts, chickpeas, salmon, or chicken are all great options.

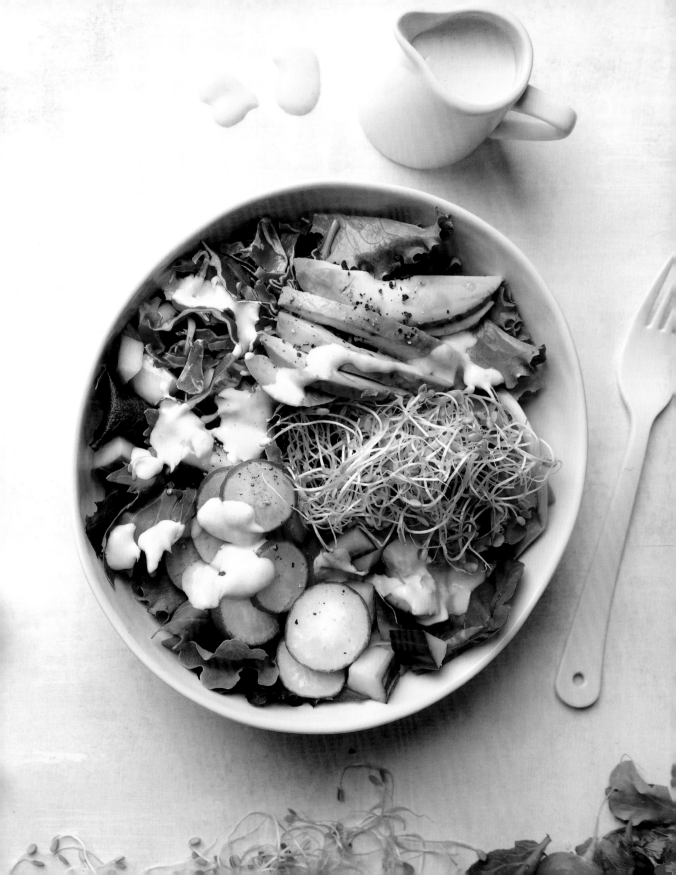

greek wedge salad
WITH BRAISED LAMB

Who doesn't love a wedge salad? We've up-leveled this Greek wedge by using romaine lettuce; drizzled it with a tangy, herbaceous red wine dressing; and topped it with our Greek-Style Braised Lamb. It's sure to be a hit with the meat lovers out there, delivering a healthy dose of dark leafy greens along with it.

Yield **4 servings**	Prep Time **15 minutes**	Cook Time **None**	**LS** CLEANSE

2 heads romaine lettuce, halved lengthwise

½ cup sliced red onion

¼ cup pitted Kalamata olives

1 English cucumber, sliced into half moons

½ cup water-packed artichoke hearts, drained and quartered

Cashew Feta (optional, page 243)

Greek-Style Braised Lamb (page 128)

For the dressing

½ cup olive oil

¼ cup red wine vinegar

1 clove garlic, minced

1 tbsp chopped fresh oregano

2 tbsp freshly squeezed lemon juice

¼ tsp Himalayan pink salt

1 To make the dressing, in a small Mason jar, combine all dressing ingredients. Secure the lid, and shake vigorously until combined.

2 To assemble the salads, place a halved romaine heart on each of four plates, and top with onion, olives, cucumber, artichokes, cashew feta, if using, and desired amount of braised lamb. Drizzle with dressing.

variation

For a meatless version, replace the lamb with Garlic and Onion Roasted Chickpeas (page 196). When not cleansing, add halved cherry tomatoes.

spicy kale caesar
WITH CRUNCHY CHICKPEAS

Although not your traditional Caesar, this cleanse-friendly, vegan variation does the trick … with a kick! Crunchy roasted chickpeas take the place of croutons, making a filling salad that can stand on its own.

Yield **1–2 servings**	Prep Time **15 minutes, plus 1-hour soak**	Cook Time **None**	CLEANSE

1 bunch kale, stems removed, chopped

Garlic and Onion Roasted Chickpeas (page 196)

For the dressing

1 cup raw cashews, soaked for at least 1 hour and drained

3 cloves garlic, chopped

1 tsp Dijon mustard

1 tsp apple cider vinegar

2 tbsp olive oil

¼ tsp Himalayan pink salt

½ tsp red pepper flakes

2 tbsp freshly squeezed lemon juice

¾ cup water

1 large celery stalk, chopped

Freshly ground black pepper, to taste

1 To make the dressing, in a high-speed blender, combine all ingredients and blend until creamy.

2 Place the kale in a large salad bowl. Add your desired amount of dressing, and toss well. Serve topped with roasted chickpeas. Leftover dressing can be stored in the refrigerator for 3 to 4 days and makes a great dip for veggies.

tip
Select whatever variety of kale looks the best or is on sale at the farmers market or grocery store.

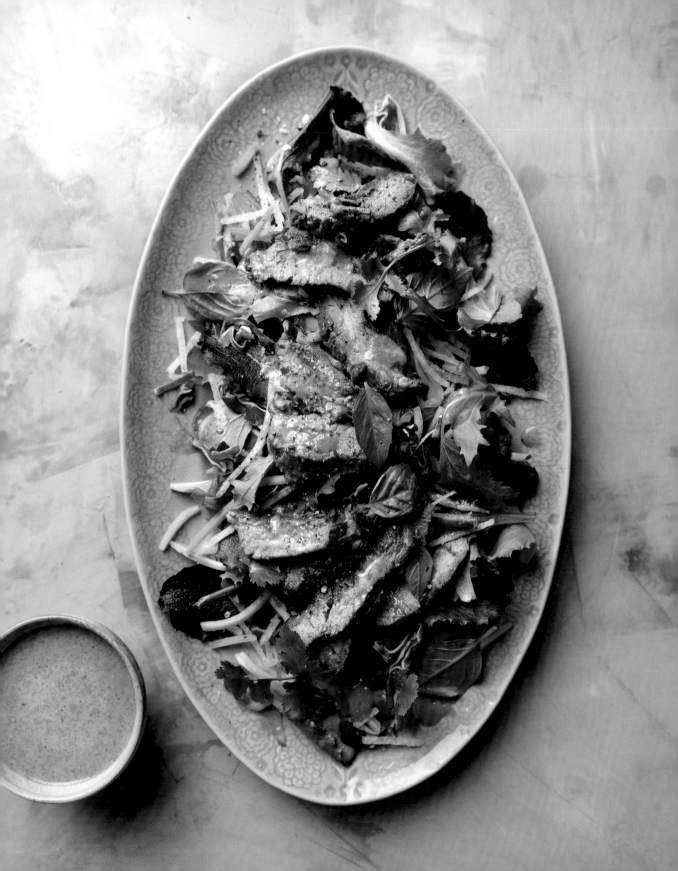

thai flank steak salad

This vibrant, family-friendly salad will make the weekly rotation with its tender steak and abundance of dark, leafy greens. You may want to make extra dressing to use as a dipping sauce for other proteins during the week—it's that good!

Yield **2-4 servings**	Prep Time **20 minutes**	Cook Time **10 minutes**	80:20

1 lb flank steak

Himalayan pink salt and freshly ground black pepper

1 tbsp olive oil

6–8 cups baby mixed greens

2 cups shredded carrots

2 cup shredded red cabbage

2 cups shredded jicama

Fresh cilantro, to garnish

Fresh Thai basil leaves (or regular basil), to garnish

For the dressing

¼ cup freshly squeezed lime juice (from about 3 limes)

2 cloves garlic, chopped

1-in piece fresh ginger, peeled and cut into chunks

¼ cup chopped fresh cilantro

½ cup chopped fresh Thai basil (or regular basil)

¼ cup olive oil

¼ cup coconut aminos

1 tbsp honey

2 tbsp fish sauce (Red Boat brand recommended)

1 Remove the steak from the refrigerator 15 to 20 minutes before cooking, and sprinkle with salt and pepper. Rub on both sides, and let it sit out to reach room temperature.

2 To make the dressing, in a high-speed blender, combine all dressing ingredients and blend until well combined. Set aside.

3 Heat a cast-iron skillet over medium-high heat. Add the oil, and heat until shimmering. Place the steak in the pan, and cook for 3 to 4 minutes per side for medium rare. (Internal temperature should be 125–130°F.)

4 Remove the steak from the pan, and transfer it to a cutting board. Let it rest for about 10 minutes. After resting, slice it thinly against the grain, ideally into strips no more than ½ inch thick. Season with additional salt and pepper, to taste.

5 To assemble the salad, top the mixed greens with equal portions of steak, carrots, cabbage, and jicama. Drizzle dressing over top, and garnish with cilantro and Thai basil. Leftover dressing can be refrigerated in an airtight glass jar for up to 1 week.

tip
Seek out 100 percent grass-fed and organic beef and bison. Many grocery stores offer meat with these certifications, or you can look online at mariposaranchmeats.com or grassrootscoop.com.

creamy vegan coleslaw

We've never been big fans of traditional coleslaw that's slathered in mayonnaise, so we knew we wanted to transform this all-American classic. Using cashews to make it creamy, this coleslaw is what nostalgic summertime dreams are made of. Perfect for a BBQ, picnic, or party, your friends will never guess that it's vegan and actually healthy!

Yield **8 servings**	Prep Time **5 minutes, plus 1-hour soak**	Cook Time **None**	CLEANSE

1 cup raw cashews, soaked for at least 1 hour and drained

⅓ cup water

½ cup roughly chopped red onion

3 tbsp apple cider vinegar

1 tbsp maple syrup

1 tsp Himalayan pink salt

¼ head red cabbage, finely shredded (about 2 cups)

¼ head green cabbage, finely shredded (about 2 cups)

2 large carrots, finely shredded

1 bunch scallions, chopped (light green and white parts only)

Freshly ground black pepper, to taste

1. In a high-speed blender, combine the cashews, water, onion, vinegar, maple syrup, and salt. Blend until smooth.

2. Place the shredded cabbages, carrots, and scallions in a large bowl. Toss with the dressing and a sprinkle of pepper, and mix well. Cover and place in the refrigerator for at least 1 hour before serving to let the flavors develop.

gut-healing slaw

Health begins in the gut. That's why you'll often find us having a tablespoon of fermented veggies (like our Vegan Kimchi) with our meals—or a big side of this bright and beautiful raw cabbage slaw. Loaded with vitamin C and insoluble fiber and topped with zinc-filled chickpea miso dressing, this one will have your gut doing a happy dance.

Yield **8 servings**	Prep Time **20 minutes**	Cook Time **None**	CLEANSE

1 medium head red cabbage, shredded very finely

3 carrots, shredded

1 cucumber, diced

1 bunch scallions, chopped (green and white parts)

1 cup chopped fresh cilantro

Himalayan pink salt and freshly ground black pepper, to taste

1 cup raw cashew halves

For the dressing

4 carrots, roughly chopped

½ white onion, roughly chopped

¼ cup chopped fresh ginger

Juice of 1 lime

2 tbsp chickpea miso (see note)

¼ cup rice vinegar

¼ cup water

2 tbsp honey

3 tbsp toasted sesame oil

2 tbsp olive oil

½ tsp Himalayan pink salt

½ tsp freshly ground black pepper

1. In a large bowl, combine the cabbage, carrots, cucumber, scallions, and cilantro. Season with salt and pepper. Set aside while you make the dressing.

2. To make the dressing, in a high-speed blender, combine all ingredients. Blend until smooth.

3. Add ¾ cup dressing to the salad, and toss to combine. Garnish with cashews just before serving. Leftover dressing can be refrigerated in an airtight container for up to 6 days.

note

We have a little love affair going on with the mighty chickpea, and that's why chickpea miso is our miso of choice. Traditional miso is made from fermented soybeans, but unless you're using certified organic soy miso, you're likely getting a genetically modified product. Plus, soy is one of the most common allergens, while chickpeas are not.

fall harvest salad
WITH APPLE CIDER VINAIGRETTE

This hearty salad is perfect for the colder months, when having a raw green salad may be less appealing. The warm, roasted butternut squash and chicken wilt the spinach perfectly, while the cinnamon and pecans whisper everything bountiful about harvest time.

Yield **2-4 servings**	Prep Time **30 minutes**	Cook Time **40 minutes**	80:20

1 small butternut squash, peeled and chopped

3 tbsp olive oil, divided

¼ tsp ground cinnamon

1 tsp Himalayan pink salt, divided

1 lb boneless, skinless chicken breasts

1 tbsp minced fresh oregano

1 tsp ground cumin

8 cups baby spinach

½ cup raw pecans, chopped

¼ cup unsweetened dried cherries

1 large pear, sliced (optional)

For the dressing
½ cup olive oil

6 tbsp apple cider vinegar

2 tbsp maple syrup

½ tsp ground cinnamon

½ tsp Himalayan pink salt

1 Preheat the oven to 400°F, and line a baking sheet with parchment paper. In a large bowl, toss the squash with 2 tablespoons oil, cinnamon, and ½ teaspoon salt. Spread evenly on the prepared baking sheet.

2 Place the chicken in a glass baking dish. Coat the chicken with the remaining 1 tablespoon olive oil, and sprinkle with the oregano, cumin, and remaining ½ teaspoon salt. Using your hands, spread the mixture over the chicken and coat well.

3 Place both the butternut squash and chicken in the oven, and roast for 25 minutes or until the squash is golden brown and the chicken is cooked through (to 165°F). The chicken will likely need an additional 10 to 15 minutes to cook after the squash comes out.

4 Meanwhile, make the dressing. In a high-speed blender, combine all ingredients. Blend until smooth.

5 Place the spinach in a large serving bowl. Top with pecans, cherries, squash, chicken, and pear slices, if desired. Drizzle with dressing, and serve.

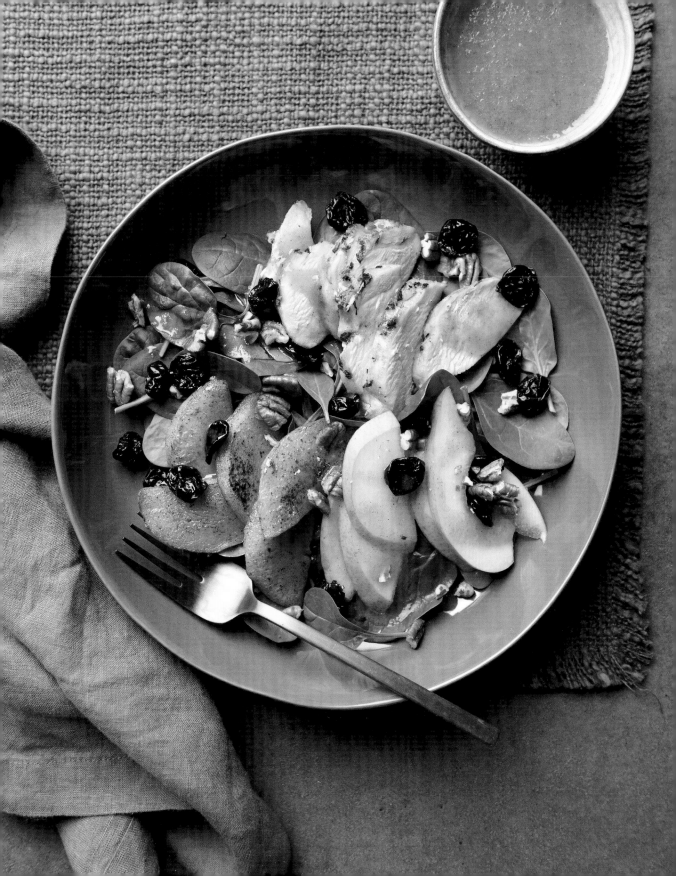

hemp seed tabbouleh

If you love tabbouleh, you're going to love this upgraded, gluten-free variation. Traditionally, tabbouleh is made with whole-grain bulgur, which contains wheat. In this version, we swapped out the bulgur for protein-packed, nutty-licious hemp seeds! Bursting with fresh herbs and lemon, this salad can be served with fresh olives, our Roasted Garlic Cauliflower Hummus, and crackers for an epic mezze platter.

Yield **4 servings**	Prep Time **15 minutes, plus 1 hour to chill**	Cook Time **None**	CLEANSE

1 cup minced fresh Italian (flat-leaf) parsley

½ cup minced fresh mint leaves

3 carrots, finely chopped

5 red radishes, finely chopped

½ cucumber, finely chopped

1 cup hemp seeds

1 tsp za'atar

2 tbsp olive oil

Juice of 2 lemons

Himalayan pink salt and freshly ground black pepper, to taste

In a large bowl, combine all ingredients and mix well. Taste and add more salt, pepper, or lemon juice, if needed. Refrigerate for at least 1 hour to let the flavors develop. Tabbouleh can be refrigerated in an airtight container for up to 2 days.

butter lettuce salad
WITH LIME FIG DRESSING

There is something so sweet and tender about butter lettuce, making it the ideal choice for a special side salad, perfect to serve while entertaining. Butter lettuces, including both Bibb and Boston varieties, are soft in texture and a little sweet—a nice alternative to the more common romaine. Make this salad to serve alongside your favorite fish or meat dish for a crowd-pleasing meal.

Yield **2–4 servings**	Prep Time **10 minutes**	Cook Time **5 minutes**	CLEANSE

¾ cup raw walnuts

Pinch of Himalayan pink salt

2 heads butter lettuce, torn into bite-sized pieces

1 bulb fennel, shaved

1 cup dried Turkish figs, stems removed, sliced

For the dressing

3 dried Turkish figs, soaked in warm water for 15 minutes and drained

3 tbsp freshly squeezed lime juice

1 tbsp apple cider vinegar

1 tbsp mirin

1 clove garlic, minced

¼ cup olive oil

Pinch of Himalayan pink salt

1 To toast the walnuts, warm a small skillet over medium-high heat. Add the walnuts and pinch of salt, and cook for about 4 to 5 minutes or until fragrant. Stir continuously, and watch closely so they don't burn. Set aside.

2 To make the dressing, in a high-speed blender, combine all ingredients. Blend until smooth and creamy. Add 1 to 2 tablespoons of warm water if needed to help with blending.

3 In a large salad bowl, toss the lettuce and fennel with desired amount of dressing. Top with figs and toasted walnuts.

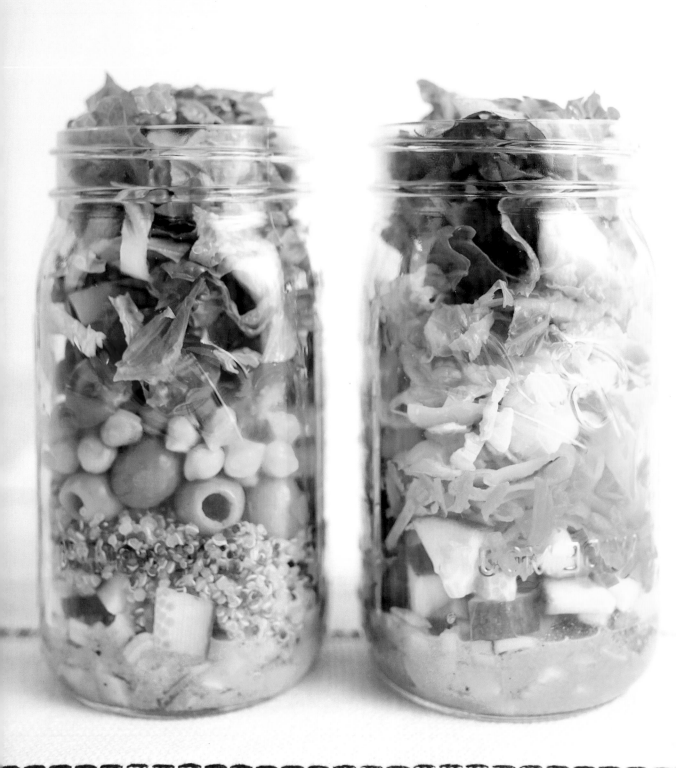

mason jar chopped salad
WITH RED WINE VINAIGRETTE

Mason jar salads are all the rage, and for good reason. Extremely versatile, colorful, and packed with fresh goodness, say hello to the perfect lunch. This Italian version is one of our favorite combinations, but the possibilities are endless. When not cleansing, try the 80:20 variation with quinoa and chickpeas. These salads will keep for up to five days in the fridge, so make a bunch in advance for the work week.

Yield **2 servings**	Prep Time **10 minutes**	Cook Time **None**	LS CLEANSE

½ red onion, diced

½ English cucumber, chopped

½ cup shredded carrots

½ cup sliced pepperoncini

½ cup quartered artichoke hearts
  (from a can or jar; packed in water)

½ head romaine lettuce, chopped

For the dressing

½ cup olive oil

¼ cup red wine vinegar

1 clove garlic, minced

1 tbsp Dijon mustard

½ tsp Himalayan pink salt

¼ tsp freshly ground black pepper

1 To make the dressing, in a small bowl, whisk together all ingredients until well combined.

2 Place two wide-mouth 32-ounce Mason jars on the counter. To each jar, add 3 tablespoons dressing. Then layer in the onion, cucumber, carrots, pepperoncini, artichoke hearts, and romaine. (Adding the ingredients in this order will prevent the veggies from getting soggy.)

3 Secure the lids on the jars to make them airtight. Refrigerate for up to 5 days.

variation

For an 80:20 version, use the same dressing, but switch up the ingredients. Omit the carrots, pepperoncini, and artichoke hearts, and replace them with cooked quinoa, chickpeas, Castelvetrano olives, and cherry tomatoes.

warm kale & beet rice salad

Move over cauliflower—beet rice is here! Warm, garlicky, and full of texture, this salad features beet as a double agent, offering both a yummy bottom and a tasty top in the form of Beet Green Pesto. We love this on its own as a meal-sized salad, but its festive colors also make it a phenomenal side dish for entertaining.

Yield **4 servings**	Prep Time **10 minutes**	Cook Time **50 minutes**	CLEANSE

2 medium beets, washed and trimmed

Pinch of Himalayan pink salt

Pinch of freshly ground black pepper

2 tbsp olive oil

4 cloves garlic, minced

2 heads lacinato kale, chopped

¼ cup roughly chopped walnuts

¼ cup **Beet Green Pesto** (page 247)

1 avocado, cubed (optional)

1 Preheat the oven to 400°F. Wrap the beets in foil, and place in the oven for about 45 minutes or until tender. Carefully unwrap and let cool. When cooled, peel and cut into quarters.

2 In a food processor, combine the beets, salt, and pepper. Pulse several times to create a rice-like consistency.

3 In a medium sauté pan, heat the oil over medium-high heat. When hot, add the garlic, kale, walnuts, and a pinch of salt. Sauté, stirring continuously, for 3 to 5 minutes or until the kale has wilted and the garlic is fragrant.

4 Add the beet rice and pesto and stir to combine. Cook for 2 minutes more, stirring occasionally. Serve warm, topped with avocado, if using.

variation

Try topping with a poached or hard-boiled egg (when not cleansing), chicken, salmon, or our Plant-Powered Not-Meat Balls (page 166).

winter roasted veggie salad
WITH MAPLE TAHINI DRESSING

There is nothing more comforting and satisfying than a zesty arugula salad topped with warm-from-the-oven roasted veggies, crisp cucumber, and cool avocado. A creamy tahini dressing unites the flavors and textures into one delicious meal-sized salad.

Yield **2–4 servings**	Prep Time **20 minutes**	Cook Time **30 minutes**	CLEANSE

4 large carrots, halved lengthwise

1 cup halved Brussels sprouts

1 bulb fennel, thinly sliced

2 tbsp olive oil

Himalayan pink salt and freshly ground black pepper, to taste

8 cups arugula

1 cup sliced English cucumber

1 avocado, sliced

For the dressing

¼ cup raw tahini (Artisana Organics brand recommended)

⅓ cup apple cider vinegar

1 tbsp freshly squeezed lemon juice

½–¾ cup water

2 tbsp maple syrup

6 tbsp olive oil

Himalayan pink salt, to taste

1 Preheat the oven to 425°F. Line a baking sheet with parchment paper or a silicone liner. Place the carrots, Brussels sprouts, and fennel on the baking sheet, and toss with the oil and a pinch of salt and pepper. Spread the vegetables evenly on the baking sheet.

2 Place the baking sheet in the oven, and roast for about 30 minutes, tossing at the half-way point to ensure even cooking. When the veggies are fork-tender, remove from the oven and season with more salt and pepper, if desired.

3 To make the dressing, in a blender or food processor, combine the tahini, vinegar, lemon juice, ½ cup water, and maple syrup. Blend until creamy. Turn the blender to low, and slowly drizzle in the oil. If the dressing is too thick, add another 2 to 4 tablespoons water to reach desired consistency. Season with salt to taste.

4 Serve the warm roasted veggies on a bed of arugula, topped with cucumber and avocado. Drizzle with dressing just before serving. Leftover dressing can be refrigerated in an airtight glass container for up to 1 week.

thai cucumber noodle salad

Thai papaya salad—typically doused in a sugary sauce—gets a major upgrade here. Cucumber noodles take the place of green papaya (which is not only difficult to find, but also presents a food-combining conundrum), making this bowl as vibrant and refreshing as they come.

| Yield **2–4 servings** | Prep Time **20 minutes** | Cook Time **5 minutes** | 80:20 |

3 English cucumbers, spiralized

3 large carrots, spiralized or julienned

1 cup halved cherry tomatoes

2 oz haricots verts (thin French green beans), trimmed

1 Thai chile, minced (optional)

½ cup chopped fresh cilantro

½ cup chopped fresh basil

¼ cup raw cashews, chopped

Pinch of red pepper flakes, or to taste

For the sauce

2 cloves garlic

2 tbsp raw cashews

¼ tsp Himalayan pink salt

¼ cup freshly squeezed lime juice

3 tbsp fish sauce (Red Boat brand recommended)

1 In a large bowl, combine the cucumbers, carrots, and tomatoes.

2 In a large saucepan with a steamer insert, steam the green beans over medium-high heat for 5 minutes. Remove from the heat and run under cold water to keep the green beans bright and crisp. Add the cooled beans to the bowl with the cucumbers, carrots, and tomatoes.

3 To prepare the sauce, in a high-speed blender, combine all ingredients. Blend until smooth.

4 Add the sauce to the prepared vegetables, and toss to combine. Divide between two bowls, and top with chile (if using), cilantro, basil, cashews, and red pepper flakes.

variation

This recipe is easily adapted to be cleanse friendly; simply omit the tomatoes. As for embellishing it 80:20 style, top it with some grilled shrimp to make it closer to the original.

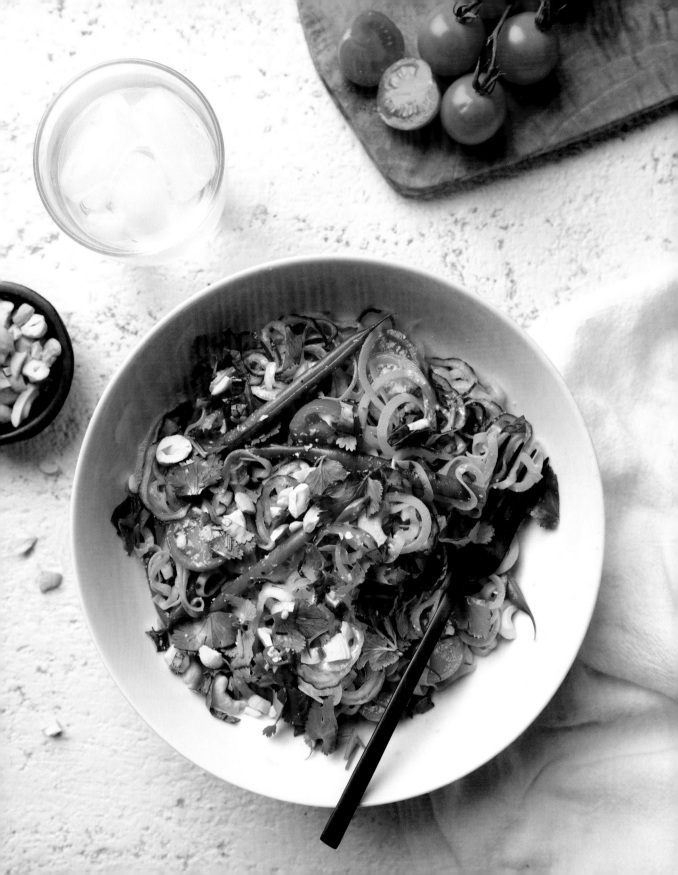

autumn wild rice salad

Wild rice, which technically is not "rice" at all, but rather the seeds of grasses grown mostly in North America, is gluten-free and chock-full of protein. This salad is a crowd-pleaser, often gracing our holiday table and perfect for potluck gatherings.

Yield **4–8 servings**	Prep Time **15 minutes**	Cook Time **45 minutes**	CLEANSE

1 cup uncooked organic wild rice, thoroughly rinsed in cold water

4 cups water

Pinch of Himalayan pink salt

1 bunch curly or lacinato kale, stems removed, finely chopped

½ bunch chard, stems removed

1 tbsp olive oil

½ bulb fennel, thinly sliced

1 bunch scallions (white and green parts), chopped

½ cup chopped fresh Italian (flat-leaf) parsley

For the dressing

½ cup olive oil

½ cup freshly squeezed lemon juice

1 garlic clove, minced

1 tsp Himalayan pink salt

1 tsp freshly ground black pepper

1 In a large pot over high heat, combine the rice, water, and salt. Bring to a boil. Once boiling, reduce to a simmer and cover, cooking until all the water is absorbed, about 45 minutes. Remove from heat, and let cool.

2 To make the dressing, in a small bowl, whisk together all dressing ingredients. Pour the dressing over the rice, and toss until fully coated.

3 To prepare the chard, stack the leaves, roll, and slice into thin ribbons. In a large bowl, combine the chard, kale, and olive oil. Using your hands, massage thoroughly until the chard and kale become soft. Add the fennel, scallions, and parsley.

4 Before serving, toss veggies and dressed rice. Season with additional salt and pepper to taste.

quinoa watercress salad

Back by popular demand, we had to share one of the best-loved recipes from our first book. Jo's parents bring this to every potluck they attend and get rave reviews every time! The watercress and fresh herbs steal the show, adding tons of flavor to this protein-packed dish. We hope you enjoy it as much as we do!

Yield **2–4 servings**	Prep Time **15 minutes**	Cook Time **20 minutes**	CLEANSE

1 cup uncooked quinoa, rinsed thoroughly

2 cups water

2 cloves garlic, minced

½ cup thinly sliced scallions (white and green parts)

2 tbsp chopped fresh mint

2 tbsp chopped fresh cilantro

1 cup chopped fresh Italian (flat-leaf) parsley

1 bunch watercress, chopped

1 cup chopped cucumber

¼ cup freshly squeezed lemon juice

¼ cup olive oil

½ cup Kalamata olives, pitted and halved

⅛ tsp Himalayan pink salt

⅛ tsp freshly ground black pepper

Pinch of red pepper flakes (optional)

1 In a large pot over high heat, combine the quinoa and water. Bring to a boil. Once boiling, reduce to a simmer and cover, cooking until all the water is absorbed, about 15 to 20 minutes. Remove from heat, and allow the quinoa to cool to room temperature.

2 Transfer the cooled quinoa to a large bowl, add the garlic and scallions, and mix well. Add the mint, cilantro, parsley, watercress, and cucumber, and stir in the lemon juice and oil. Add the olives, and season with salt, pepper, and red pepper flakes, if using. Let sit for at least 30 minutes before serving to allow the flavors to blend.

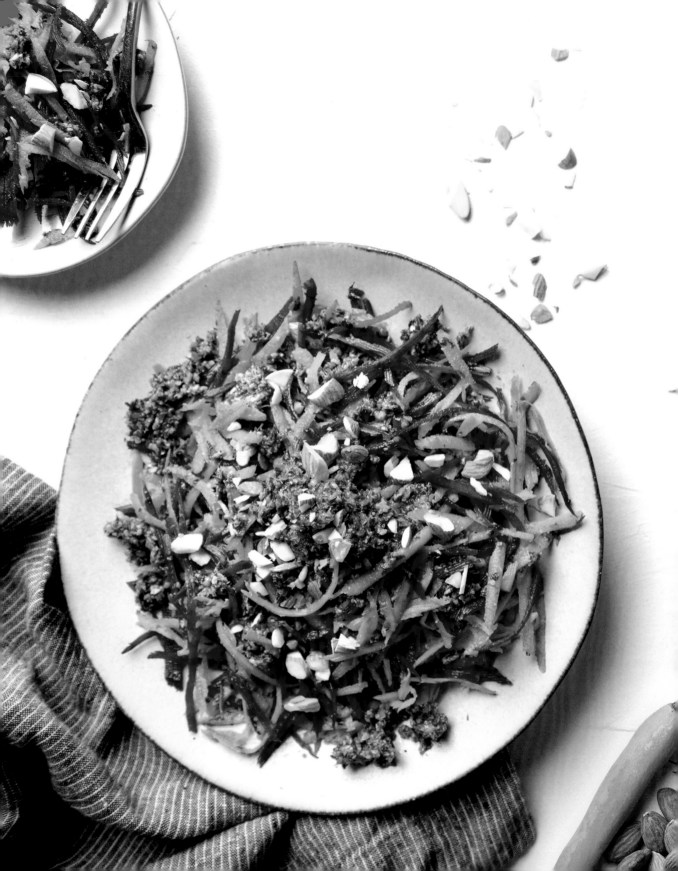

carrot top pesto salad

We love pesto. It's a staple in our kitchens—the perfect dip for some veggies or topper for a piece of fish. Here we wanted to make a colorful side salad that would utilize the "double agent" carrot—a vegetable with a tasty top as well as a yummy bottom. This delicious, vividly hued salad is just one way to experiment with different types of herbs or greens and nuts or seeds for pesto.

Yield **4 servings**	Prep Time **15 minutes, plus 4-hour soak**	Cook Time **None**	**LS** CLEANSE

1 bunch organic carrots with green tops, roughly chopped (reserve the green tops for pesto)

2 beets, peeled

Juice of 1 lemon

For the pesto
Greens from 1 bunch organic carrots, thoroughly washed (see note)

1 clove garlic, peeled

¼ cup raw almonds or sunflower seeds, soaked for 4 hours, drained and rinsed

⅓ cup olive oil

¼ tsp Himalayan pink salt

Freshly ground black pepper, to taste

1. In a food processor fitted with a shredding blade, shred the carrots and beets. (A box grater works, too.) Transfer the shredded beets and carrots to a medium bowl, and toss with lemon juice. Set aside.

2. To make the pesto, fit the food processor with the chopping blade, and add the carrot greens, garlic, and almonds or sunflower seeds. Pulse a few times to break up the ingredients. With the food processor running, slowly drizzle in the oil until the mixture is emulsified but still has some texture. Add salt and pepper, and pulse once more.

3. Add ¾ of the pesto mixture to the shredded carrot and beet mixture. Toss to coat. Serve salad with remaining pesto on the side.

note
This recipe is best with vibrant carrot greens fresh from the farmers market.

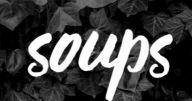

soups

chicken bone broth 108

veggie broth 109

cleansing ginger beet soup 110

healing vegetable congee 112

veggie kelp noodle pho.. 113

golden soup 115

purification soup 116

slow cooker butternut lentil soup 117

slow cooker bison stew 118

superfood green "soup" 120

nightshade-free turkey chili 121

vietnamese chicken pho.. 123

chicken bone broth

Bone broth is a staple for vibrant health and our go-to whenever anyone in the family starts to feel under the weather. Use it as a base for your soups, or sip throughout the day. Made in the slow cooker from organic bones and veggies, this flavorful elixir promotes healthy skin and helps to heal the gut. Easily adaptable, it can be made with whatever fresh veggies and herbs you have on hand.

| Yield **2 quarts** | Prep Time **10 minutes, plus 1-hour soak** | Cook Time **24 hours** | CLEANSE |

1 cooked chicken carcass (about 1½ lb)

10 cups filtered water

1 tbsp apple cider vinegar

1 large onion, quartered

10 cloves garlic, smashed

2 cups roughly chopped organic vegetables (carrots, celery, mushrooms, parsnips, zucchini, leeks, etc.)

2 tbsp chopped fresh herbs (rosemary, sage, thyme, oregano, etc.)

½ tsp Himalayan pink salt, or to taste

½ tsp freshly ground black pepper

⅛ tsp cayenne pepper (optional)

1-in piece fresh ginger, sliced (optional)

Juice of ½ lemon

Large handful of fresh Italian (flat-leaf) parsley, chopped

1 After removing all edible meat from the chicken, put the bones, skin, and connective tissues in a large slow cooker. Add water to cover the bones. Add the apple cider vinegar, cover, and let soak for at least 1 hour.

2 Add the onion, garlic, vegetables, herbs, salt, pepper, cayenne, and ginger, if using, to the bones and water. Set the slow cooker to Low, cover, and cook for 24 hours or at least overnight. As the broth cooks, skim off any foam that forms on the surface. The liquid will reduce; add more water if the level drops a lot.

3 In the last 30 minutes of cooking, add the lemon juice and parsley. Taste and adjust seasoning, if needed. When the broth is done, remove the lid and allow it to cool. Following food safety precautions, make sure the broth has cooled to 70°F within 2 hours.

4 When the slow cooker is cool to the touch, strain the broth through a fine sieve and/or cheesecloth to remove the bits of bone, vegetables, and herbs. Refrigerate.

5 Once chilled, a layer of fat may form at the surface. This fat helps the broth stay fresh longer and can be scraped off or used in other cooking. If there's enough gelatin in the broth, it may turn into a jelly, which is great! To reconstitute, simply heat the jelly in a saucepan, adding a bit of water, if desired, to thin. Broth will keep in the refrigerator for 5 to 6 days, and it can be frozen up to 4 months.

variation

To make on the stove top, soak the bones as directed in a large stock pot. Bring the broth to a boil over high heat, then reduce heat to low, and simmer for at least 8 hours.

veggie broth

Once you get into the habit of making your own homemade broth, you'll never go back. It's so easy to make, either on the stove top or in a multicooker, such as an Instant Pot. Delicious as a warming beverage on a cold day or as the base for one of our healing soups, it's a great staple to have on hand in the freezer.

Yield **2 quarts**	Prep Time **10 minutes**	Cook Time **2 hours (stove top) or 40 minutes (multicooker)**	CLEANSE

1–2 onions, unpeeled, quartered

2–3 carrots, unpeeled, cut into 2-in pieces

3–4 stalks celery, cut into 2-in pieces

4–5 sprigs fresh thyme

1 bay leaf

1 small bunch Italian (flat-leaf) parsley

1 tsp whole peppercorns

1 cup shiitake mushrooms

1 clove garlic

1-in piece fresh ginger, unpeeled

1 tsp ground turmeric

Himalayan pink salt (optional), to taste

stove top instructions

1   Place all ingredients, except salt, in a large stock pot. Add filtered water to cover vegetables by 2 to 3 inches.

2   Bring the mixture to a boil over high heat. When boiling, reduce the heat to a simmer, and cook for 1 to 2 hours. Taste and season with salt, if using.

3   Strain through a fine mesh strainer, and discard solids. Broth can be refrigerated in an airtight container for up to 1 week or frozen for up to 2 months.

multicooker instructions

1   Place all ingredients, except salt, in a multicooker. Add filtered water to cover. Close and lock the lid. Turn the venting knob to the sealing position. Select Pressure (high) for 15 minutes.

2   When cook time is complete, allow the pressure to naturally release for 15 to 20 minutes and then manually release the remaining pressure. Taste and season with salt, if using.

3   Strain through a fine mesh strainer, and discard solids. Broth can be refrigerated in an airtight container for up to 1 week or frozen for up to 2 months.

 tip

If you make juice at home, save the leftover vegetable pulp for making broth. Simply reserve the pulp from your kale, collards, parsley, cilantro, carrots, and celery, and stick it in the freezer. (Avoid cucumber, lemon, or fruit pulp.) When it's time to make veggie broth, add the frozen pulp in place of or in addition to some fresh veggie scraps.

cleansing ginger beet soup

Beets are inherently anti-inflammatory and detoxifying, making this earthy soup perfect for cleansing. They're also known to boost stamina and aid in circulation while oxygenating the blood. We hope you love this beautifully vibrant soup, with its healthy dose of warming ginger, as much as we do.

Yield **4 servings**	Prep Time **15 minutes**	Cook Time **55 minutes**	LS CLEANSE

4 medium beets, peeled, trimmed, and chopped

1 leek, roughly chopped

1 bulb fennel, roughly chopped (about 1 cup)

2 cloves garlic, roughly chopped

3-in piece fresh ginger, peeled and roughly chopped

8 cups water

Sea salt and freshly ground black pepper, to taste

Juice of 1 lemon

1 tbsp chopped fresh chives, to garnish

1 In a large stock pot, combine the beets, leek, fennel, garlic, ginger, and water. Bring to a boil over high heat. When boiling, reduce heat to a simmer. Cook for about 45 minutes or until the beets are fork-tender. Let cool for 5 to 10 minutes.

2 Transfer the soup to a high-speed blender, and blend on high until smooth. Taste and season with salt and pepper. Add the lemon juice and chives just before serving.

tip

The top portion of the beetroot, called beet greens, can (and should!) be eaten. Discard them, and you lose out on one of the best dark leafy greens out there. We love to rotate them into our green smoothies, adding more iron than even our beloved spinach.

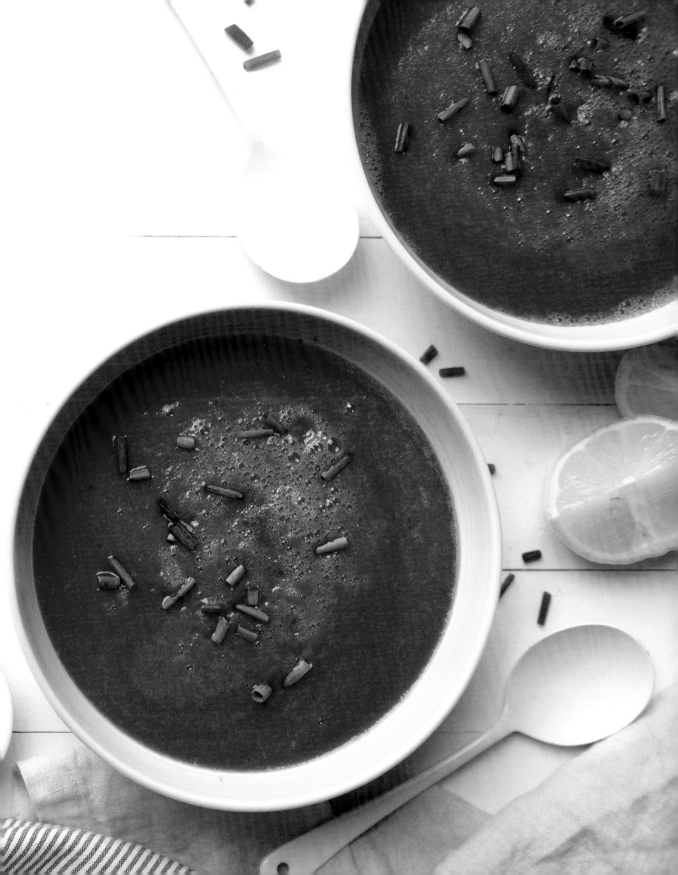

healing vegetable congee

Congee is a traditional healing food in Chinese medicine that is easy on digestion. We created our version of congee at the request of one of our star health coaches, Jessica, who often recommends it to cleansers who struggle with gas and bloating. Although often enjoyed for lunch or dinner, it's perfectly suitable for breakfast, too. We choose to keep it vegan, but feel free to swap in bone broth for extra digestive support.

Yield **2 servings**	Prep Time **15 minutes**	Cook Time **80 minutes**	CLEANSE

2 tbsp olive oil

½ cup thinly sliced scallions (white and green parts)

2-in piece fresh ginger, peeled and thinly sliced

2 large cloves garlic, thinly sliced

1 tsp ground turmeric

½ cup uncooked short-grain brown rice, rinsed

5 cups **Veggie Broth** (page 109) or low-sodium vegetable broth

1 tsp Himalayan pink salt

Freshly ground black pepper, to taste

3 medium carrots, diced

¾ cup sliced shiitake mushrooms

1 bunch lacinato kale, stems removed, cut into ribbons

¼ cup chopped fresh cilantro, to garnish

1 In a small Dutch oven, heat the oil over medium heat. Add the scallions, ginger, and garlic, and stir for 2 minutes or until fragrant. Add the turmeric and brown rice, and stir to combine. Add the vegetable broth, salt, and pepper. Bring to a boil, reduce heat to low, and simmer, covered. Cook for about 1 hour, stirring often.

2 When the rice is cooked and the mixture thickens, add the carrots and mushrooms, cover, and continue cooking for 10 minutes. When the carrots are tender but still firm, add the kale, stir to combine, cover, and cook an additional 8 to 10 minutes. Taste and adjust salt and pepper to your liking. You can also add more vegetable broth for a more soup-like consistency. Serve garnished with cilantro.

variation

If not cleansing, top the congee with a hard-boiled egg or shredded chicken.

veggie kelp noodle pho

When we created our Vietnamese Chicken Pho, we loved it so much that we knew we needed a veggie version. This recipe features a ginger-infused broth that's loaded with veggies and calls for both kelp and zucchini noodles. Nourishing and oh-so-healing, this slurpable soup is vibrancy in a bowl.

Yield **2 servings**	Prep Time **20 minutes**	Cook Time **30 minutes**	CLEANSE

2 star anise pods

4 whole cloves

2 cinnamon sticks

¼–½ tsp red pepper flakes, or to taste

4 cloves garlic, smashed

¼ cup sliced ginger

6 cups **Veggie Broth** (page 109) or low-sodium vegetable broth

¼ cup coconut aminos

1 tbsp olive oil

2 large portobello mushrooms, chopped

Pinch of Himalayan pink salt

1 (12oz) package kelp noodles, soaked in warm water for 15 minutes and drained

1 medium zucchini, spiralized

1 cup shredded carrots

To garnish

2 tbsp chopped fresh Thai basil

Handful of fresh mint leaves

2 tbsp sliced scallions

½ cup fresh bean sprouts

1 lime, sliced

1. In a dry medium stock pot or Dutch oven, heat the star anise, cloves, cinnamon sticks, and red pepper flakes over medium-high heat for about 30 seconds or until the spices are fragrant.

2. Add the garlic, ginger, vegetable broth, and coconut aminos. Bring to a boil over high heat, then reduce heat to simmer. Cover and cook for 30 minutes.

3. While the broth simmers, in a medium sauté pan, heat the oil over medium heat. When hot, add the mushrooms and salt. Cook, stirring frequently, for 4 to 6 minutes. Remove from heat and set aside.

4. Using a sieve and a large bowl, carefully strain the broth, discard the spices, and transfer the broth back to the pot or Dutch oven.

5. To assemble the pho, place about 1 cup kelp noodles in each of two bowls. Equally divide the zucchini noodles, carrots, and mushrooms between the two bowls and top with warm broth. Garnish with basil, mint, scallions, and bean sprouts. Serve with lime to squeeze over top.

variation

If not cleansing, top with a hard-boiled egg.

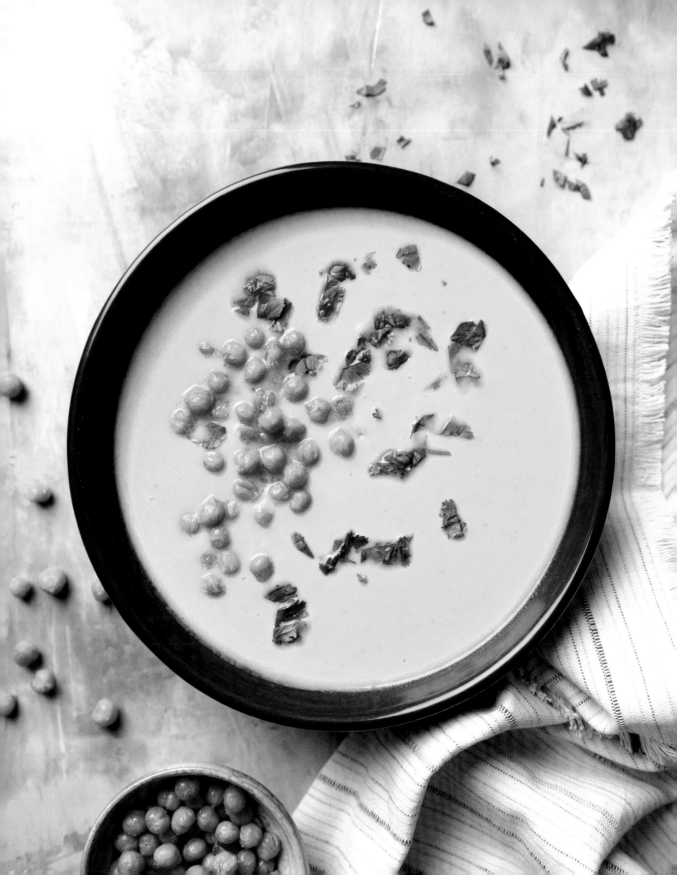

golden soup

We love bright and colorful food, and this soup is no exception. Featuring turmeric, a spice known for its anti-inflammatory properties, this soup is rich, creamy, and oh-so-grounding. Like the popular Curried Carrot Soup from our previous book, this is cleanse friendly, easy on digestion, and quick to prepare.

Yield **4–6 servings**	Prep Time **15 minutes**	Cook Time **30 minutes**	CLEANSE

2 tbsp olive oil

2 tsp yellow curry powder

1 tsp ground turmeric

1 head cauliflower, cut into florets (5–6 cups)

4 medium stalks celery, chopped

1 yellow onion, chopped

2 cloves garlic, chopped

1 tsp Himalayan pink salt, divided

3 cups **Veggie Broth** (page 109) or low-sodium vegetable broth

1 (13.5oz) can full-fat coconut milk

2 tbsp freshly squeezed lemon juice

Freshly ground black pepper, to taste

Finely chopped fresh cilantro (optional), to garnish

Garlic and Onion Roasted Chickpeas (optional, page 196), to garnish

1 In a medium saucepan, heat the oil, curry powder, and turmeric over low heat, stirring frequently, for 2 minutes. Stir in the cauliflower, celery, onion, garlic, and ½ teaspoon salt, and toss to coat. Cook, stirring frequently, for 10 minutes.

2 Stir in the vegetable broth and coconut milk. Bring to a boil, and then reduce heat to low. Simmer for 10 minutes or until the vegetables are very tender. Remove from heat, and cool for at least 1 minute.

3 In a high-speed blender, working in batches of no more than 2 cups, purée the soup. Return the soup to the pot, and heat through. Season with lemon juice, remaining ½ teaspoon salt, and pepper. Serve topped with cilantro and roasted chickpeas, if using.

variation
To make this Purification friendly, omit the chickpeas and coconut milk. Add an extra 1½ cups vegetable broth to thin as desired. This soup is also great for the Low Sugar Track without the chickpeas.

purification soup

This soup is perfect for Purification while on the Conscious Cleanse or anytime you're under the weather. A twist on the beloved Bieler's Broth from our previous book, here we added a head of roasted garlic for its potent medicinal properties, as well as Swiss chard, an often overlooked but powerful dark leafy green.

| Yield **4 servings** | Prep Time **10 minutes** | Cook Time **50 minutes** | **CLEANSE** |

1 head garlic

3 tsp olive oil, divided

1 yellow onion, chopped

1 cup chopped celery

1 medium zucchini, chopped

1 bunch Swiss chard, stems removed, roughly chopped

4 cups **Veggie Broth** (page 109) or low-sodium vegetable broth

½ cup fresh Italian (flat-leaf) parsley, packed

Freshly squeezed lemon juice, to serve

1 Preheat the oven to 400°F. Slice ¼ to ½ inch from the top of the garlic head, exposing the individual cloves. Place the garlic head cut side up on a piece of foil, drizzle with 1½ teaspoons oil, and rub the oil into the exposed cloves. Seal the foil around the garlic.

2 Place the foil-wrapped garlic on a baking sheet cut side up. Place in the oven, and roast for 35 minutes. Remove from the oven, unwrap the garlic and let cool. When the garlic is cool to touch, squeeze out the cloves.

3 In a large stock pot, warm the remaining 1½ teaspoons oil over medium-high heat. Add the onions, and sauté for about 5 minutes or until translucent, stirring occasionally. Add the celery, zucchini, and Swiss chard. Cook for 5 minutes more, stirring occasionally. Add the roasted garlic cloves and vegetable broth, increase the heat, and bring to a boil. When boiling, reduce heat to low and simmer, covered, for 15 minutes.

4 Remove from heat and let cool, uncovered. When cool, transfer the soup to a blender. Add the parsley, and blend until smooth, working in batches if necessary. Serve warm with a squeeze of lemon.

slow cooker butternut lentil soup

Nothing beats the feeling of coming home to a warm, nutrient-dense, hearty soup. Lentils are a great source of plant-based protein, making this slow cooker soup one of our favorites for meatless Monday. Just toss everything into the slow cooker and go. Now that's the way to kick off the week!

| Yield **4–8 servings** | Prep Time **15 minutes** | Cook Time **6 hours (high); 8 hours (low)** | 80:20 |

2 cups cubed butternut squash

2 cups diced celery (about 4 stalks)

1 large yellow onion, diced

3 cloves garlic, minced

1 cup green lentils, rinsed

1 (15oz) can diced tomatoes

4 cups **Veggie Broth** (page 109) or low-sodium vegetable broth

2 tsp ground turmeric

1½ tsp ground cumin

½ tsp ground cinnamon

1 tsp Himalayan pink salt

½ tsp freshly ground black pepper

1 (13.5oz) can full-fat coconut milk

3 cups kale, stems removed, cut into ribbons

Juice of ½ lemon

Pinch of red pepper flakes (optional)

1 Place the butternut squash, celery, onion, garlic, lentils, tomatoes, vegetable broth, turmeric, cumin, cinnamon, salt, and pepper in a slow cooker. Cover and set to Low for 7 to 8 hours or High for 5 to 6 hours.

2 In the last 15 minutes of cooking, stir in the coconut milk and kale, and replace the lid. Cook until the kale is wilted. Ladle into bowls and garnish with fresh lemon juice and red pepper flakes, if using.

slow cooker bison stew

Surprised to see stew on a cleanse? We intentionally made this cleanse friendly for those of you who like a heartier meal, swapping out potatoes for parsnips and beef for the more sustainably raised bison. This robust stew is one for the whole family—cleansing or not.

Yield **4 servings**	Prep Time **15 minutes**	Cook Time **8 hours (slow cooker) or 1 hour (multicooker)**	CLEANSE

2 tbsp coconut oil

2 yellow onions, chopped

4 cloves garlic, minced

4 carrots, chopped

4 stalks celery, chopped

2 parsnips, chopped

1 lb bison, cut into 1-in cubes

2 bay leaves

1 tsp Himalayan pink salt

1 tsp freshly ground black pepper

2–4 cups low-sodium beef broth (Pacific Foods brand recommended) or homemade beef stock

1 tbsp arrowroot powder

1–2 tbsp finely chopped Italian (flat-leaf) parsley, to garnish

variation

If you do not have time to turn the stew to High for the last hour of cooking in the slow cooker, you can put the stew in a pot on the stove and bring it to a simmer. Add the arrowroot, and stir constantly until thickened.

slow cooker instructions

1 In a sauté pan, heat the oil over medium heat until melted. Add the onions and garlic, and cook for 5 minutes. Transfer onions and garlic to a slow cooker.

2 Add the carrots, celery, parsnips, bison, bay leaves, salt, and pepper to the slow cooker. Pour 4 cups broth over all the ingredients. The liquid should cover the vegetables and meat; add more broth or water to cover if needed. Place the lid on the slow cooker, and cook for 6 to 8 hours on Low.

3 During the last hour, increase the heat to High. In a small bowl, mix the arrowroot powder with 2 tablespoons water until it is broken down into a paste. Add the arrowroot mixture to the stew, and stir until thickened. Remove the bay leaves. Serve hot, topped with parsley.

multicooker instructions

1 Set a multicooker to Saute (normal). Add the oil. When melted, add the onions and cook for 3 minutes, stirring regularly. Add the garlic, and cook for 2 minutes more. Then add the carrots, celery, parsnips, bison, salt, and pepper, and mix together. Add the bay leaves and 2 cups broth.

2 Press Cancel to end the sauté setting. Lock the lid in place with the vent in the sealing position. Set to Pressure (high) for 35 minutes.

3 When time is up, allow natural release for at least 15 minutes before manually releasing the sealing valve. In a small bowl, mix the arrowroot powder with 2 tablespoons water until it is broken down into a paste. Add the arrowroot mixture to the stew, and stir until thickened. Remove the bay leaves. Serve hot, topped with parsley.

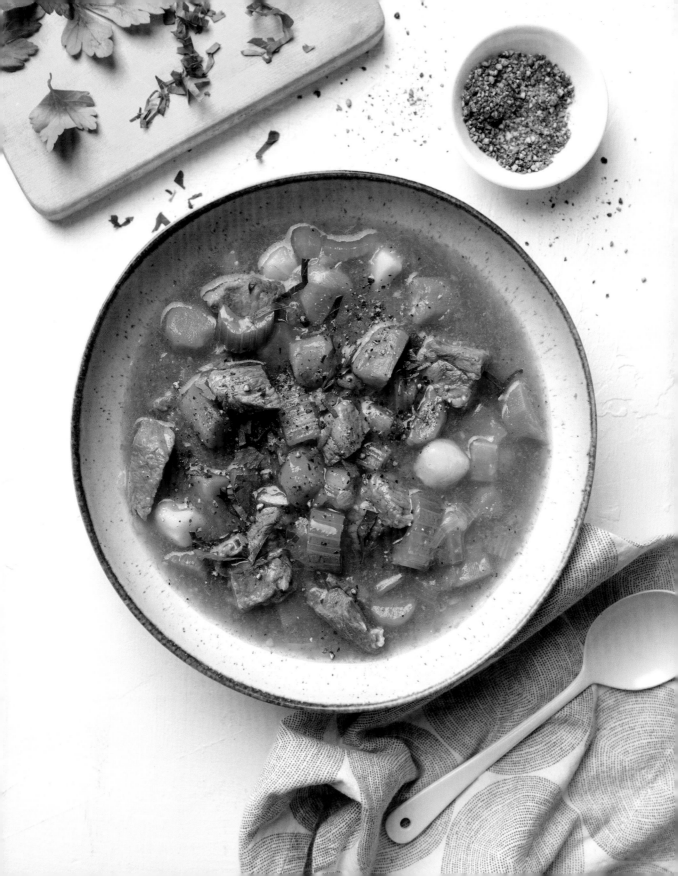

superfood green "soup"

Perfect for our Low Sugar Track, this green "soup" is like a blended salad, a savory alternative to a green smoothie. Loaded with live enzymes, alkalizing greens, and fresh herbs, this raw "soup" has endless potential. Enjoy it in a bowl with a spoon, or sip it out of a mug for maximum nourishment.

Yield **1–2 servings**	Prep Time **10 minutes**	Cook Time **None**	**LS** CLEANSE

1 medium zucchini, chopped

3 stalks celery, chopped

1 bulb fennel, chopped

1 cup spinach

1 lemon, peeled

1 avocado

1 cup water

½ tsp Himalayan pink salt

In a high-speed blender, combine all ingredients. Blend until smooth. Enjoy!

tip

Craving something warm and cozy? Blend this "soup" on high for 2 minutes to create a warmer soup.

nightshade-free turkey chili

With no tomatoes or peppers, this is not your mom's traditional chili. Instead, we use golden beets and carrots along with bone broth and fresh oregano to make the perfect cleanse-friendly winter meal. This chili freezes well, so make a double batch and keep some on hand for a quick meal another time.

Yield **4–6 servings**	Prep Time **20 minutes**	Cook Time **45 minutes**	CLEANSE

1 tbsp olive oil

1 medium yellow onion, diced

2 stalks celery, diced

4 carrots, diced

1 medium golden beet, peeled and diced

4 cloves garlic, minced

4 cups **Chicken Bone Broth** (page 108) or low-sodium chicken stock (Pacific Foods brand recommended), divided

2 tbsp minced fresh oregano, plus more to garnish

1 tsp onion powder

½ tsp garlic powder

¼ tsp ground cinnamon

⅛ tsp ground ginger

2 tsp Himalayan pink salt

1 medium head cauliflower, cut into florets

2 lb ground turkey

1 In a large stock pot, heat the oil over medium-high heat. When hot, add the onions, celery, carrots, and beet. Cook for about 7 minutes or until the onions are translucent.

2 Add the garlic and cook, stirring, for 3 minutes or until garlic is fragrant. Add 3 cups bone broth, oregano, onion powder, garlic powder, cinnamon, ginger, and salt. Bring to a boil, and then reduce heat to medium-low, cover, and simmer for 20 minutes.

3 Meanwhile, in a pot with a steamer basket, steam the cauliflower for about 10 minutes or until fork-tender. Transfer the cauliflower to a high-speed blender, and add the remaining 1 cup bone broth. Blend until smooth. Set aside.

4 In a large, nonstick skillet, cook the turkey over medium-high heat, stirring frequently, for about 5 minutes or until browned.

5 Add the cooked turkey and the cauliflower purée to the pot with the vegetables, and simmer, covered, for an additional 15 minutes. Garnish with fresh oregano, if desired, before serving.

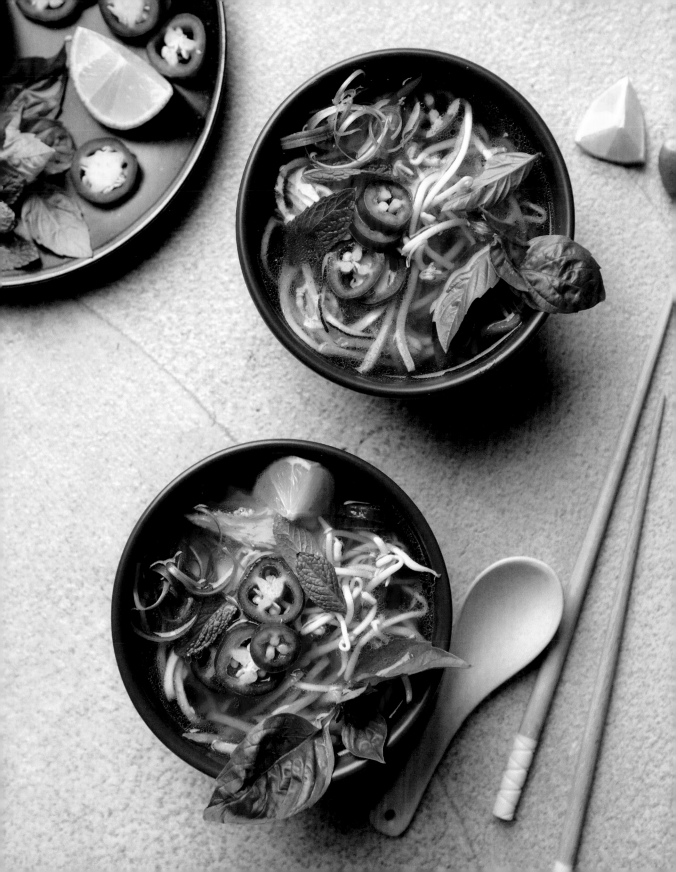

vietnamese chicken pho

Pho is a Vietnamese soup that typically consists of broth, rice noodles, herbs, and meat. Our version features a delicious ginger-infused broth over zucchini noodles, giving this pho more nutrient bang for your buck. It's perfect if you're craving Asian food but want to skip take-out—and the bloat!

Yield **2 servings**	Prep Time **15 minutes**	Cook Time **25 minutes**	CLEANSE

2 tbsp olive oil

¼ cup peeled and minced fresh ginger

4 pods star anise

1 tsp ground coriander

½ tsp red pepper flakes

4 cups **Chicken Bone Broth** (page 108) or low-sodium chicken stock (Pacific brand recommended)

2 large skinless, boneless chicken breasts

¼ cup fish sauce (Red Boat brand recommended)

2 tsp honey

Himalayan pink salt and freshly ground black pepper, to taste

2 medium zucchini, spiralized

To serve

2 cups shredded carrots

2 tbsp chopped fresh Thai basil

Handful of fresh mint leaves

½ cup sliced scallions

½ cup fresh bean sprouts

½ jalapeño, thinly sliced (optional)

1 lime, cut into wedges

1   Set a multicooker (such as an Instant Pot) to Saute (normal) and add the oil to the pot. When hot, add the ginger and cook, without stirring, for about 4 minutes or until slightly charred. Add the star anise, coriander, and red pepper flakes. Cook for 1 minute more or until fragrant.

2   Add the chicken broth to the pot along with the chicken, fish sauce, and honey. Secure the lid. Cancel sauté mode, and select Pressure (high) for 15 minutes. When done, turn off the multicooker and allow the pressure to naturally release for 10 minutes. After 10 minutes, turn the valve to quick release any remaining pressure.

3   Remove the chicken from the pot. Strain the broth and season with salt and pepper to taste. Skim some of the fat from the broth.

4   When the chicken is cool enough to handle, shred it and divide between two large soup bowls. Add zucchini noodles and broth to each bowl, and top with carrots, basil, mint, scallions, bean sprouts, jalapeño, if using, and lime wedges.

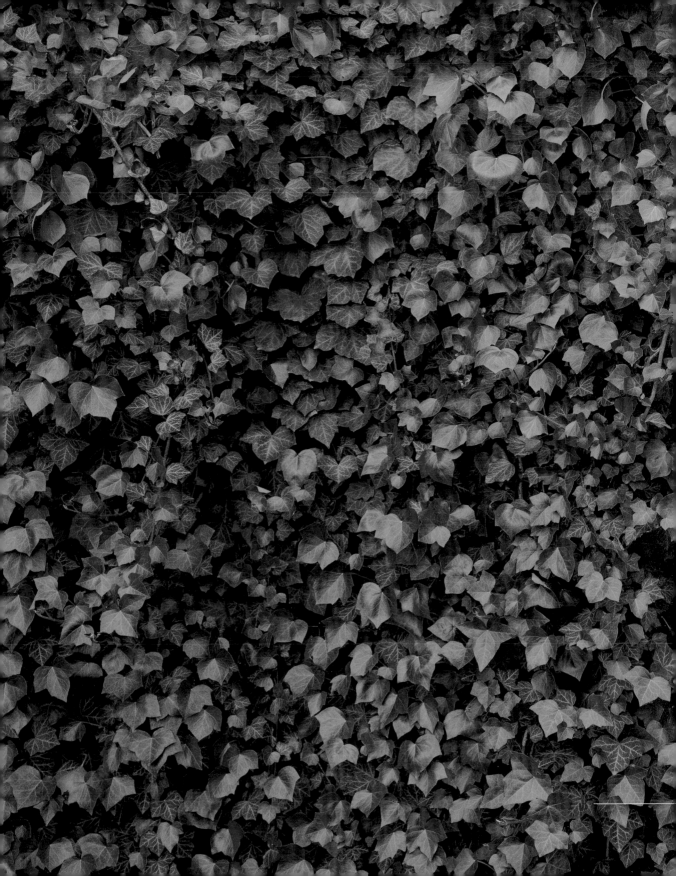

meat & seafood

slow cooker lamb tagine 126

greek-style braised lamb 128

lamb gyro lettuce wrap 129

bison broccoli stir-fry 130

bison bolognese 132

herb & cashew crusted chicken............................133

honey mustard chicken skewers...........................134

cashew chicken stir-fry 135

grilled chicken 137

dry rub chicken wings 138

curry chicken salad..139

shrimp pad thai 140

ginger scallion turkey burgers 142

chipotle lime salmon 143

coconut glazed halibut 145

ahi tuna poke bowl...146

salt & pepper snapper 147

ginger salmon bowl..148

steamed sea bass 150

sweet miso black cod..151

easy weeknight fish tacos 153

slow cooker lamb tagine

As busy moms and business owners, we know firsthand how challenging dinnertime can be. Getting something healthy, quick, and tasty on the table after a long day can be stressful. But not anymore—slow cooker, to the rescue! This Moroccan-inspired dish is loaded with flavor and color—perfect for a chilly night.

Yield **6 servings**	Prep Time **10 minutes**	Cook Time **8 hours**	80:20

2 tsp ras el hanout (see note)

¾ tsp smoked paprika

1 tsp grated fresh ginger

2 cloves garlic, chopped

1 tbsp coconut oil

1 lb boneless lamb shoulder, cut into 1-in pieces

Himalayan pink salt and freshly ground black pepper

2 cups chicken or vegetable stock

1 medium onion, finely diced

3 carrots, cut into 1-in pieces

½ delicata squash, peel on, seeds removed, cut into 1-in pieces

½ lemon, seeds removed, cut into small pieces

1 bunch cilantro stems (bottom portion of the bunch), finely chopped, plus leaves for garnish

½ cup pitted green olives, rinsed

Cauliflower rice or steamed kale (optional), to serve

½ cup unsweetened dried cherries (optional), to garnish

1 In a medium skillet, toast the ras el hanout and smoked paprika over medium heat until fragrant. Add to a slow cooker along with the ginger and garlic.

2 In the same skillet, heat the oil over medium heat until it is melted and the pan is hot. Season the lamb with salt and pepper. Add to the skillet, and brown on each side. Add to the slow cooker.

3 Add a splash of chicken or vegetable stock to the skillet to deglaze the pan, scraping any browned bits from the bottom. Pour the stock into the slow cooker.

4 Add the onion, carrots, squash, lemon, cilantro stems, olives, and remaining stock to the slow cooker. Stir to combine.

5 Cover and cook on Low for 8 hours or until the lamb is fork-tender and the liquid has reduced. Season to taste with salt and pepper.

6 Serve over cauliflower rice or steamed kale, if using. Garnish with cilantro leaves and dried cherries, if using.

note

Ras el hanout is a Moroccan spice blend that can be found in the spice section of gourmet grocers.

variation

To make this recipe cleanse friendly, simply omit the delicata squash or use another hardy vegetable, like parsnips, turnips, or Brussels sprouts, in its place.

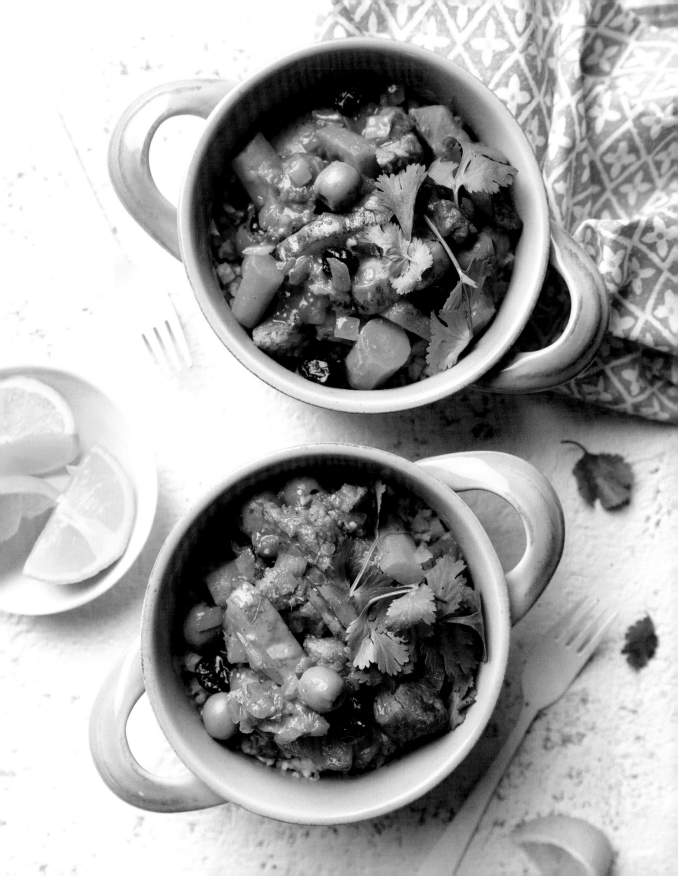

greek-style braised lamb

Grass-fed lamb is leaner and healthier than grain-fed beef. This tender lamb dish, flavored with garlic and fresh oregano, is perfect for a warming winter meal or anytime you want an easy dinner with little prep, thanks to the multicooker. Enjoy the leftovers in a wrap or on our Greek Wedge Salad.

Yield **4 servings**	Prep Time **10 minutes**	Cook Time **60 minutes**	CLEANSE

1 tbsp olive oil

2 lb lamb shoulder roast

¼ cup chicken broth

1 tbsp stone ground mustard

5 cloves garlic, peeled and smashed

¼ cup chopped fresh oregano

½ tsp Himalayan pink salt

¼ tsp freshly ground black pepper

2 tbsp freshly squeezed lemon juice

1 Set a multicooker to Saute (normal). When hot, add the oil and sear the lamb on both sides, about 45 to 60 seconds per side.

2 In a small bowl, whisk together the broth, mustard, garlic, oregano, salt, pepper, and lemon juice. Add to the pot with the lamb, and stir to coat. Select Meat/Stew mode for 45 minutes.

3 When the cook time is complete, allow the pressure to release naturally for 10 minutes before manually venting.

tip

To make this in a slow cooker, first sear the lamb on all sides in a sauté pan on the stove top. Transfer to a slow cooker with the rest of the ingredients, and cook on Low for 8 hours.

lamb gyro lettuce wrap

Jules' boys love a good flavor-filled gyro! Here we use romaine lettuce as the perfect stand-in for pita bread. Stuffed with succulent braised lamb and plenty of veggies, it's great for lunch on the go.

Yield **1 serving**	Prep Time **15 minutes**	Cook Time **None**	CLEANSE

6 large romaine lettuce leaves

¼ cup finely chopped baby spinach

¼ English cucumber, sliced (about 8 slices)

⅓ red onion, thinly sliced

¼ cup pitted Kalamata olives

¼ cup halved artichoke hearts (from a jar or can, packed in water)

½ cup **Greek-Style Braised Lamb** (page 128)

½ cup **Green Tzatziki Sauce** (page 245)

1 To make the wrap, lay a piece of parchment paper on a cutting board or work surface. Layer the romaine leaves horizontally in the center of the parchment paper to create a lettuce base 8 to 9 inches wide.

2 Fill the wrap by spreading out the spinach, and then layer on the cucumber, onion, olives, artichokes, and lamb. Spread evenly across the romaine leaves, leaving room at the outside edges for rolling your wrap in step 3. Top with green tzatziki sauce.

3 When you have all your fillings in place, starting at the end closest to you, roll the lettuce wraps burrito-style, as tightly as possible, using the parchment paper as your base.

4 Halfway through rolling, tuck the ends of the wrap toward the center, and then continue to roll the lettuce wrap, keeping the parchment paper as taut as possible.

5 Cut the wrap in half and then wrap in another piece of parchment paper, and refrigerate until ready to eat.

note

Creating a romaine wrap in parchment paper is not as hard as it sounds. Think deli-style wrap or your standard sub shop method. With practice, you'll get the hang of this and be so glad you did. These wraps are the perfect to-go lunch, and the filling combinations are endless.

bison broccoli stir-fry

Beef and broccoli is a favorite Chinese takeout order for many people, so we knew we had to make a cleanse-friendly, up-leveled version. Simple and oh-so-delicious, this is the perfect weeknight dinner.

| Yield **4 servings** | Prep Time **10 minutes** | Cook Time **15 minutes** | **CLEANSE** |

1 lb bison skirt steak, cut into thin strips (see note)

1 head broccoli, cut into florets

1 tbsp avocado oil

2 cloves garlic, minced

2-in piece fresh ginger, peeled and finely chopped

Pinch of Himalayan pink salt

2 cups halved cremini or button mushrooms

Cauliflower rice or sautéed greens (optional), to serve

Sesame seeds (optional), to garnish

For the marinade

1 tbsp toasted sesame oil

2 tbsp coconut aminos

1 tsp arrowroot powder

½ tsp Himalayan pink salt

¼ tsp freshly ground black pepper

For the stir-fry sauce

2 tbsp coconut aminos

1 tbsp fish sauce (Red Boat brand recommended)

2 tsp toasted sesame oil

¼ tsp freshly ground black pepper

1. To make the marinade, in a small bowl, whisk together sesame oil, coconut aminos, arrowroot powder, salt, and pepper. In a shallow baking dish, toss the bison with the marinade to coat, and place in the refrigerator for 20 minutes.

2. To make the stir-fry sauce, in a small bowl, whisk together the coconut aminos, fish sauce, sesame oil, and pepper. Set aside.

3. In a pot with a steamer insert, steam the broccoli over medium-high heat for 5 minutes or until the broccoli is tender but still crisp. Remove from heat and run cold water over to keep bright and crisp. Set aside.

4. In a large, cast-iron skillet, heat the avocado oil over high heat. When the pan is hot, reduce the heat to medium, and add the garlic and ginger. Season with a pinch of salt, and cook for about 10 seconds or until fragrant.

5. Increase the heat to medium-high, and add the marinated bison. (Discard any excess marinade.) Spread the meat evenly over the bottom of the skillet, and cook for about 4 minutes or until the edges of the bison are slightly darkened and crispy. Flip and do the same on the other side.

6. Add the stir-fry sauce and mushrooms, and cook for 2 to 3 minutes or until browned. Add the broccoli, toss to combine, and cook for another 30 seconds. Serve hot over cauliflower rice or sautéed greens, if using, and garnish with sesame seeds, if using.

note

You can ask your butcher to cut the bison into 1-inch, bite-sized strips.

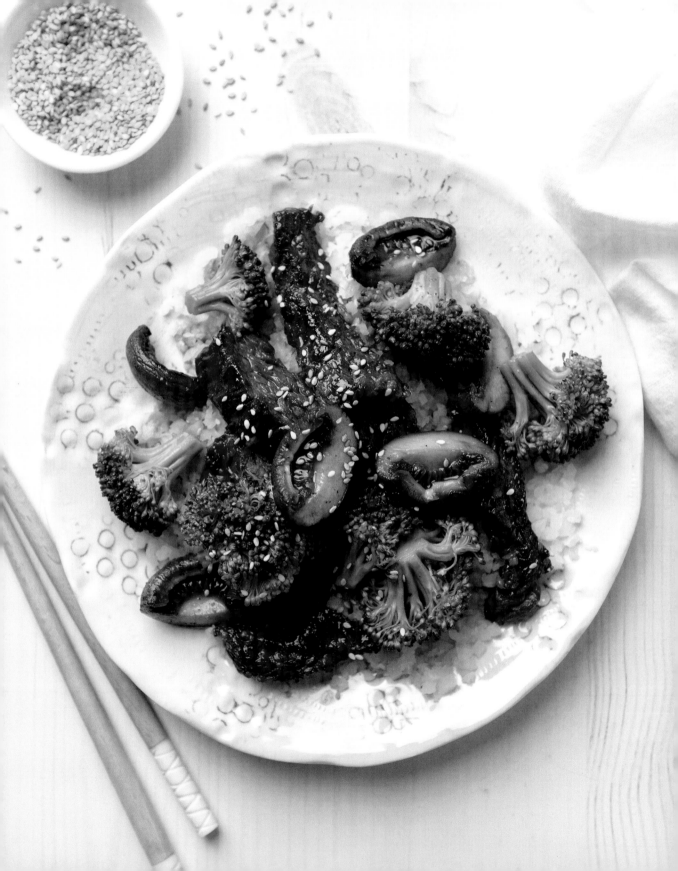

bison bolognese
WITH ZUCCHINI NOODLES

The first time Jo's daughter tried this recipe, she licked the bowl clean! Zucchini noodles make it cleanse friendly and veggie-forward, but you could also use spaghetti squash, chickpea pasta, or rice pasta (when not cleansing). Because the sauce is a bit labor-intensive, make a big batch and freeze some for later use.

Yield **4 servings**	Prep Time **5 minutes**	Cook Time **25 minutes**	**LS** CLEANSE

2 tbsp olive oil, divided

1 lb ground bison

2 cups **No-Mato Marinara** (page 244)

2 cloves garlic, minced

6 medium zucchini, spiralized

Himalayan pink salt and freshly ground black pepper, to taste

Fresh basil, finely chopped (optional), to garnish

1 Heat a large skillet over high heat. When hot, add 1 tablespoon oil and the bison. Stir and cook for about 5 minutes or until the meat is browned and no longer pink. Stir in the marinara sauce. Bring to a low boil, reduce the heat to low, and simmer for 15 minutes.

2 Meanwhile, in a separate skillet, heat the remaining 1 tablespoon oil over medium heat. Add the garlic, and sauté for 30 seconds. Add the zucchini noodles, and cook for about 5 minutes, stirring occasionally, until soft. Season with salt and pepper.

3 To serve, divide the zucchini noodles among four plates and top with your desired amount of bolognese. Garnish with basil, if using.

 tip
The No-Mato Marinara can be made ahead and refrigerated in an airtight glass container for up to 7 days.

herb & cashew crusted chicken
WITH LEMONY ARUGULA

This healthy twist on breaded chicken is a staple in Jo's family. In place of traditional breading, we've blended up a mix of fresh herbs and cashews to make a gluten-free, grain-free coating that's crunchy and full of flavor. And the best part is, you can have it on the table in just 30 minutes!

Yield **4 servings**	Prep Time **15 minutes**	Cook Time **30 minutes**	

4 boneless, skinless chicken breasts

½ cup chopped fresh Italian (flat-leaf) parsley

2 tbsp minced fresh thyme

2 tbsp minced fresh rosemary

½ cup raw cashews, finely chopped or pulsed in food processor

½ tsp Himalayan pink salt

¼ tsp freshly ground black pepper

2 tbsp Dijon mustard

2 tbsp olive oil

8 handfuls of arugula

2 tsp freshly squeezed lemon juice, or more to taste

1 Using a meat tenderizer, pound the chicken breasts to an even thickness, about ½ inch thick. In a small bowl, mix the parsley, thyme, rosemary, cashews, salt, and pepper. Spread the herb and cashew mixture on a plate.

2 Coat each chicken breast with Dijon mustard and then press in the herb mixture to coat.

3 In a large skillet, heat the oil over medium heat. Working in batches if needed, cook the chicken for 3 to 4 minutes per side or until fully cooked.

4 In a large bowl, toss the arugula with lemon juice to taste. Serve the chicken on a bed of dressed arugula.

honey mustard chicken skewers

Want to simplify your weeknight dinner plan? Make this sheet pan dinner. This kid-friendly favorite is easy to prepare ahead of time—plus, eating food on a stick is just more fun! Try it with our Parsnip Fries.

Yield **4 servings**	Prep Time **20 minutes, plus 1 hour to marinate**	Cook Time **25 minutes**	CLEANSE

2 lb boneless, skinless chicken breasts, cut into 2-in cubes

2 medium zucchini, cut into ½-in rounds

12 small button mushrooms

1 red onion, quartered

For the marinade

¼ cup olive oil, divided

3 tbsp honey

2 tbsp Dijon mustard

4 cloves garlic, minced

1 tsp dried oregano

1 tsp dried basil

1 tsp Himalayan pink salt

½ tsp freshly ground black pepper

1. To make the marinade, in a small bowl, whisk together all ingredients.

2. Place the chicken in a shallow baking dish, and coat with half of the marinade. Place the zucchini, mushrooms, and onion in a large bowl, and toss to coat with the remaining marinade. Place the chicken and vegetables in the refrigerator to marinate for at least 1 hour.

3. Place 8 to 10 skewers in water to soak for 10 minutes. Preheat the oven to 450°F. Line a baking sheet with parchment paper.

4. Assemble the chicken skewers by placing chicken pieces on each skewer. Prepare vegetable skewers by alternating among zucchini, mushrooms, and onions. Slide about 8 pieces onto each skewer, being careful to leave enough room to handle the skewers comfortably. You will wind up with 4 chicken and 4 veggie skewers.

5. Place the skewers on the prepared baking sheet, and season with additional salt and pepper, if desired. Bake for 25 minutes, turning skewers once halfway through cooking.

cashew chicken stir-fry

We love a good stir-fry! Loaded with colorful veggies and tossed with the perfect savory sauce, this is the quintessential weeknight meal. If you're like us and obsessed with cashews and Asian-inspired flavors of sesame, ginger, and garlic, you'll love this one.

Yield **4 servings**	Prep Time **15 minutes**	Cook Time **15 minutes**	LS 80:20

2 tbsp olive oil

1 small sweet yellow onion, sliced (about 1 cup)

1 lb boneless, skinless chicken breast, cut into 1-in chunks

1 red bell pepper, sliced

2 carrots, peeled and julienned

1 head broccoli, cut into small florets (about 2 cups)

1 cup snow peas or snap peas

2 scallions, thinly sliced (green and white parts)

¾ cup raw cashews

4–6 cups cauliflower rice, warmed, to serve

For the sauce

½ cup vegetable or chicken broth

½ cup coconut aminos

2 tbsp fish sauce (Red Boat brand recommended)

4 tsp toasted sesame oil

2 tsp minced garlic

2 tsp minced fresh ginger

½–1 tsp red pepper flakes (see note)

1 To make the sauce, in a small bowl, whisk together all ingredients until well combined. (Adjust red pepper flakes to taste.) Set aside.

2 In a large skillet, warm the olive oil over medium-high heat. Add the onion and chicken, and cook for 5 to 6 minutes.

3 Add the bell pepper and carrots, and cook for 3 to 4 minutes. Add the broccoli and snow peas, and cook for 1 to 2 minutes more, stirring continuously. Add the scallions, cashews, and stir-fry sauce, and continue to stir and cook for another 2 to 3 minutes. Serve hot over warm cauliflower rice.

note

If you like heat, go for the full teaspoon of red pepper flakes. To make this kid friendly, use ½ teaspoon in the sauce, and reserve the other half to adjust the spice once served.

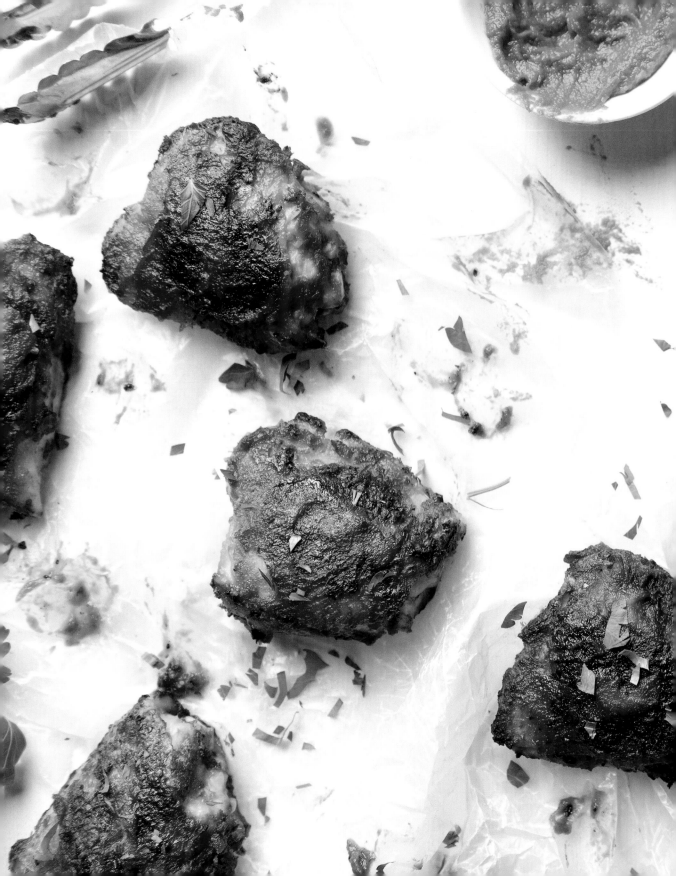

grilled chicken
WITH TOMATO-FREE BBQ SAUCE

BBQ grilled chicken is an American classic, and now you have a cleanse-friendly version. Made with our tomato-free, no-sugar BBQ sauce, it's so smoky and delicious, you'll never miss the original.

Yield **4–6 servings**	Prep Time **15 minutes**	Cook Time **1 hour**	**LS** CLEANSE

3 lb chicken thighs and legs, skin on and bone in

Himalayan pink salt

2 tbsp chopped fresh Italian (flat-leaf) parsley, to garnish

For the sauce

1 beet, scrubbed and trimmed

1 tbsp olive oil

1 cup diced onion

1 cup diced carrot

1 tbsp freshly squeezed lemon juice

5 tbsp apple cider vinegar

2 tbsp blackstrap molasses

1 tbsp minced fresh ginger

1 clove garlic, crushed

½ tsp smoked salt

1. To make the sauce, preheat the oven to 375°F. Wrap the beet loosely in foil and place in the oven. Roast for 1 hour or until soft. Remove the beet from the oven, remove the foil, and set aside to cool. When the beet has cooled, peel off the skin. (It should slip off easily.) Cut the peeled beet into quarters and set aside.

2. In a medium saucepan, heat the oil over medium heat. Add the onion and carrots, and sauté until onion is translucent, about 5 minutes. Remove from heat.

3. In a high-speed blender, combine the roasted beet, cooked onion and carrots, lemon juice, vinegar, molasses, ginger, garlic, and smoked salt. Blend until smooth. Transfer the mixture to a large saucepan, and simmer for 15 minutes to thicken.

4. Season the chicken with Himalayan pink salt on both sides. Preheat a gas grill to medium-low heat (about 300°F). Place the chicken on the heated grill, and cook for about 30 minutes with the lid closed, turning occasionally. Before the chicken is fully cooked, brush BBQ sauce over the surface every 3 to 5 minutes until the chicken reaches an internal temperature of 165°F. When the chicken is cooked through, remove the chicken from the grill and let it rest for 10 minutes. Garnish with parsley.

tip

The BBQ sauce can be made ahead and refrigerated in an airtight glass container for up to 7 days.

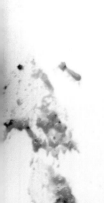

dry rub chicken wings

Chicken wings are usually synonymous with greasy bar food, to which many of our cleansers' partners (ours included) would say, "Yum!" These cleanse-friendly, grilled wings deliver all the yum without the unhealthy trans fats—spicy, smoky, and finger-licking good.

Yield **4 servings**	Prep Time **5 minutes, plus 30 minutes to marinate**	Cook Time **16 minutes**	CLEANSE

2 lb chicken wings

2 tbsp olive oil

3 cloves garlic, minced

½ tsp cayenne pepper

1 tsp dried oregano

1 tsp dried rosemary

1 tsp hot chili powder

1 tsp Himalayan pink salt

1　In a large, resealable plastic bag, combine all ingredients and shake to coat the chicken in oil and seasonings. Place in the refrigerator to marinate for at least 30 minutes.

2　Preheat a grill to medium heat. Lightly oil the grates with olive oil, and place the wings on the grill. Close the grill lid, and cook for 8 minutes on each side. Enjoy hot!

curry chicken salad

Jo's husband, Adam, developed this recipe as a healthy alternative for their daughter. Most chicken salads have eggs, preservatives, and dairy. This recipe is gluten-, dairy-, and sugar-free and gets its sweetness from raisins and a little monk fruit sweetener. It's great in a lettuce wrap or over a green salad.

Yield **4 servings**	Prep Time **10 minutes**	Cook Time **15 minutes**	80:20

1½ tsp olive oil

1 lb boneless, skinless chicken thighs

1 tbsp freshly squeezed lemon juice

1 tsp curry powder

½ cup vegan mayonnaise (Sir Kensington's brand recommended)

½ tsp Himalayan pink salt

1 tsp Lakanto Classic Monkfruit Sweetener or honey (optional)

3 stalks celery, minced

½ cup chopped raw cashews

⅓ cup raisins

Freshly ground black pepper, to taste

1 In a large pan, heat the oil over medium heat. When hot, add the chicken thighs. Cook for 15 minutes or until they are no longer pink, turning once. Set aside to cool.

2 Meanwhile, in a medium bowl, combine the lemon juice, curry powder, mayonnaise, salt, and sweetener, if using. Mix well. Add the celery, cashews, and raisins.

3 When the chicken is cool, dice into small pieces. Add the chicken to the mayonnaise mixture, and stir well. Taste and adjust pepper and other seasonings as needed.

shrimp pad thai

We love Asian food but stopped ordering takeout long ago in favor of homemade recipes like this one—clean and fresh, with spiralized taro root in place of rice noodles. You'll never miss the real thing. Taro is similar to potato in taste and full of fiber and resistant starch, which can help balance your blood sugar.

Yield **4 servings**	Prep Time **15 minutes**	Cook Time **10 minutes**	80:20

1½ lb taro root, peeled and spiralized

16 medium shrimp, peeled and deveined

Himalayan pink salt and freshly ground black pepper

1 tbsp olive oil

¾ cup sliced scallions

1 clove garlic, minced

8 cups baby spinach

For the sauce

1 tbsp chickpea miso

1 tbsp raw tahini (Artisana Organics brand recommended)

1 tbsp coconut aminos

2 tsp freshly grated ginger

2 tbsp unsweetened rice vinegar

2 tsp maple syrup

1 tsp chili paste or sriracha sauce

Dash of ground cinnamon

1½ tbsp water

To garnish

Black or white sesame seeds

Fresh cilantro leaves

Lime wedges

1. In a large saucepan of salted, boiling water, cook the spiralized taro root for about 5 minutes or until tender but firm. (Thinner spirals will cook more quickly.) Drain in a colander and set aside.

2. Pat the shrimp dry. Season with salt and pepper and set aside.

3. To make the sauce, in a small bowl, combine all ingredients. Whisk until smooth.

4. In a large saucepan, heat the oil over medium heat. When hot (but not smoking), add the shrimp, scallions, and garlic. Sauté for 1 to 2 minutes. Add the drained taro root and the sauce, and toss until combined. Cook for 3 to 4 minutes more or until the noodles are heated through and the shrimp turns pink. (Be careful not to overcook, as the shrimp will become tough and the taro will become sticky.)

5. Serve over a bed of baby spinach, and garnish with sesame seeds, cilantro, and lime wedges.

variation

If you are unable to find taro root, you can substitute zucchini noodles.

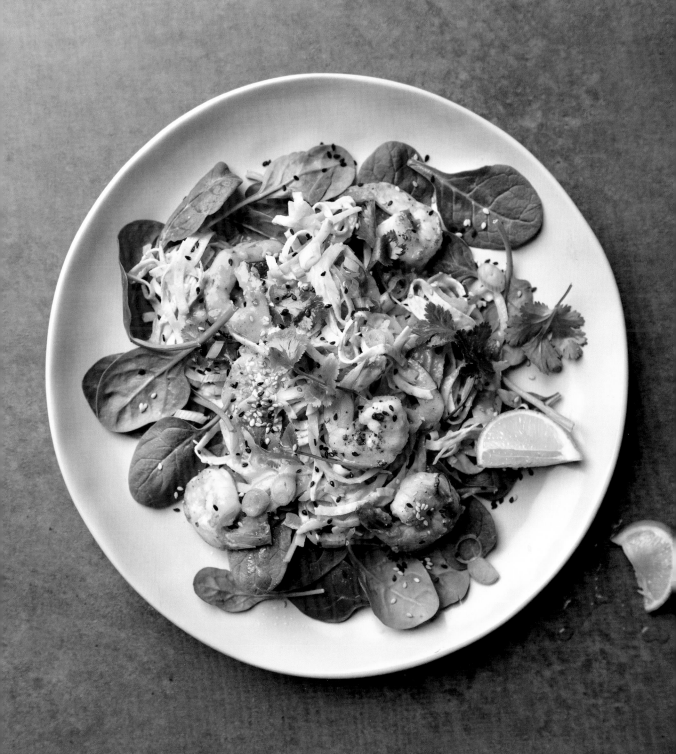

ginger scallion turkey burgers

The turkey burger recipe in our first book is a cleanser favorite, so we knew we had to do another one. If you like ginger, you'll love this recipe for flavorful turkey patties. Instead of a bun, try serving it on a lettuce wrap topped with our Egg-Free Avocado Mayo and Vegan Kimchi.

Yield **12 mini burgers**	Prep Time **10 minutes**	Cook Time **30 minutes**	

1 lb ground turkey breast

1 lb ground turkey thigh

1 tbsp olive oil

½ cup chopped sweet white onion

2 tbsp grated fresh ginger

2 scallions, minced (green and white parts)

½ cup chopped fresh cilantro

1½ tsp Himalayan pink salt

¼ tsp freshly ground black pepper

To serve (optional)

Lettuce leaves

Egg-Free Avocado Mayo (page 245)

Vegan Kimchi (page 242)

1 Preheat the oven to 375°F. Line a baking sheet with foil.

2 In a large bowl, use your hands to combine the turkey (breast and thigh meat), oil, onions, ginger, scallions, cilantro, salt, and pepper.

3 Form the mixture into 12 patties (3–4oz each) and place on the prepared baking sheet. Bake for 30 minutes, turning once.

4 Serve on a lettuce "bun" topped with avocado mayo and kimchi, if using.

chipotle lime salmon
WITH MASSAGED KALE

This quick and healthy salmon dish is one of our favorites—simple, delicious, and packed with anti-inflammatory omega-3s. We cook this salmon on the grill, making cleanup that much easier.

Yield **2 servings**	Prep Time **10 minutes**	Cook Time **20 minutes**	**LS** CLEANSE

1 lb wild-caught salmon

3 tbsp olive oil, divided

Juice and zest of 1 lime

1 tsp chipotle powder

1 tsp Himalayan pink salt, divided

1 bunch kale, stems removed, chopped

Juice of ½ lemon

½ avocado, sliced

1 Preheat the grill to medium-high heat. Drizzle the salmon with 2 tablespoons oil and lime juice; sprinkle with lime zest, chipotle powder, and ½ teaspoon salt. Place the salmon on the grill, skin side down, for 15 to 20 minutes or until cooked through.

2 In a large bowl, combine the kale, lemon juice, and remaining 1 tablespoon oil and ½ teaspoon salt. Using your hands, massage the kale thoroughly until it becomes soft.

3 Cut the salmon into the desired number of pieces and serve over the kale, topped with avocado slices.

tip

If you don't have a grill, you can broil the salmon. Preheat the broiler to medium, and position an oven rack 3 to 4 inches from the heat source. Place the salmon skin side down in a shallow baking dish and drizzle with 2 tablespoons oil and lime juice; sprinkle with lime zest, chipotle powder, and ½ teaspoon salt. Broil for 6 to 8 minutes, basting with the remaining marinade once or twice during cooking.

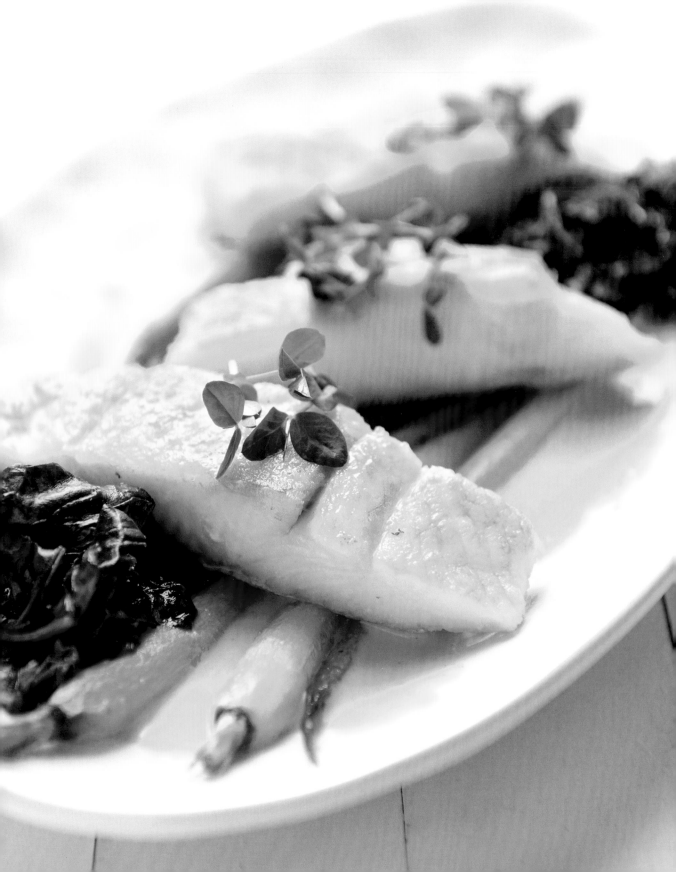

coconut glazed halibut
WITH BUTTERNUT CURRY SAUCE

An all-time favorite in the Conscious Cleanse community, this recipe is sure to impress your guests! Halibut, high in brain-boosting omega-3 fatty acids, pairs beautifully with the flavorful, warming curry sauce.

Yield **4 servings**	Prep Time **15 minutes**	Cook Time **40 minutes**	80:20

4 tbsp coconut oil, divided

½ yellow onion, roughly chopped

2 cups cubed butternut squash

2 tsp yellow curry powder

1 (13.5oz) can full-fat coconut milk

Himalayan pink salt, to taste

2 large bunches Swiss chard, stems removed, roughly chopped

2 tbsp coconut aminos

4 (4oz) halibut fillets, skin on (see note)

To serve (optional)
Microgreens or pea tendrils
Reduced balsamic vinegar
Roasted carrots

1 To make the sauce, in a medium skillet, heat 2 tablespoons oil over low heat. Add the onions and butternut squash, and cook until the squash is tender but not very brown, stirring frequently. Stir in the curry powder and coconut milk. Carefully transfer the squash mixture to a blender. Purée until creamy. Taste and add salt as needed. Set aside.

2 In a large pan, heat 1 tablespoon oil over medium heat. Add the chard and sauté until wilted and tender. Finish with coconut aminos, adding more to taste. Set aside.

3 Heat a cast-iron or nonstick skillet over medium-high heat. Season the halibut with salt on each side. Add the remaining 1 tablespoon oil to the pan, and swirl to coat. Place the halibut in the pan skin side down. Cook for 5 minutes, flip fish, and cook for another 3 minutes or until fish is opaque in the center.

4 To assemble, place a generous portion of the butternut sauce on a plate followed by a heap of chard. Top with halibut and microgreens, balsamic, and roasted carrots, if using.

note
Sometimes halibut can be hard to find. Feel free to substitute your favorite whitefish in place of the halibut if needed.

ahi tuna poke bowl

Although tuna is not a go-to fish for us on the cleanse, Jules' family loves a good poke bowl once in a while. Simply put, a poke bowl is deconstructed sushi. We use cauliflower rice as our base to simplify digestion, but you could easily swap it out for brown rice for a more traditional poke bowl.

| Yield **4 servings** | Prep Time **15 minutes** | Cook Time **10 minutes** | 80:20 |

1 lb sushi-grade ahi tuna, cut into ¾-in cubes

1 head cauliflower, cut into florets (about 3½ cups)

1 tbsp avocado oil

2 ripe avocados, sliced

¼ cup sliced scallions (green and white parts)

½ cup microgreens, to garnish

For the marinade

¼ cup coconut aminos

1½ tsp brown rice vinegar

2 tsp toasted sesame oil

¼ tsp red pepper flakes, or to taste

1 In a medium bowl, combine all marinade ingredients. Add the tuna, and gently toss. Set aside while you prepare the cauliflower rice and other bowl ingredients.

2 To make the cauliflower rice, in a food processor, pulse the cauliflower florets to a rice-like consistency. In a large skillet over medium heat, warm the avocado oil and cauliflower rice. Stir continuously until warm, about 5 to 10 minutes.

3 Divide the cauliflower rice evenly among four bowls, and top each bowl with equal portions of the tuna mixture, avocado, and scallions. Garnish with microgreens.

variation

Replace the cauliflower rice with an equal amount of cooked brown rice.

salt & pepper snapper

The fresh, bold flavor of this snapper hits the spot. Shallot, garlic, and parsley coat the fish to give it an herbaceous, green "crust." This is a great cleanse friendly, weeknight dish the entire family will enjoy.

| Yield **4 servings** | Prep Time **10 minutes, plus 20 minutes to marinate** | Cook Time **10 mintues** | CLEANSE |

4 (6–8oz) thick red snapper fillets (check for pinbones and remove with tweezers before cooking)

1 tbsp olive oil

4 lemon wedges, to garnish

For the marinade

4 tbsp olive oil

2 cloves garlic, minced

1 shallot, finely minced

½ cup chopped fresh Italian (flat-leaf) parsley

Juice and zest of 2 lemons

1½ tsp Himalayan pink salt

1½ tsp freshly ground black pepper

1 To make the marinade, in a small bowl, whisk together all ingredients. Set aside.

2 Place the fish in a shallow glass baking dish, and pour about ¾ cup marinade over top (reserve the rest for serving). Place in the refrigerator to marinate for 20 minutes.

3 To ensure that the fish cooks evenly and that the skin remains crispy and delicious, score the fillets. Using a sharp knife, make shallow cross-hatched cuts on the skin of each fillet just before searing.

4 In a large skillet, heat 1 tablespoon oil over medium heat until hot but not smoking. Place the fish in the pan skin side down, and cook for 5 to 7 minutes or until you can lift the fish from the pan without sticking. Flip carefully and cook for 3 to 4 minutes more or until fish is cooked through. Drizzle the remaining marinade over top of the fish and serve with lemon wedges to garnish.

variation

Rockfish, called the "poor man's snapper," makes a good alternative for this recipe if red snapper isn't available.

ginger salmon bowl

If you had any doubts about the magic of vibrancy bowls, this one is sure to wow. Featuring ginger salmon piled high on a mound of arugula and loaded with fresh veggies, this is a bowl of all our favorite things.

Yield **4 servings**	Prep Time **20 minutes**	Cook Time **20 minutes**	CLEANSE

1 lb asparagus, trimmed

½ tsp olive oil

¼ tsp Himalayan pink salt

1 lb wild-caught salmon, cut into 4 pieces

8 cups arugula

2 cups finely shredded red cabbage

1 English cucumber, cut in ¼-in rounds

2 avocados, sliced

2 nori sheets, torn into pieces

For the dressing

¼ cup freshly squeezed lemon juice

2 cloves garlic, minced

2-in piece fresh ginger, minced or grated

2 tbsp olive oil

½ tsp Himalayan pink salt

1 Preheat the oven to 400°F, and line a baking sheet with parchment paper.

2 To make the dressing, in a small bowl, whisk together all ingredients.

3 Place the asparagus on the prepared baking sheet, and toss with oil and salt. Place the salmon fillets between the asparagus, and drizzle 1 tablespoon dressing over the salmon. Bake for 15 to 20 minutes or until the salmon flakes easily with a fork. Remove from the oven.

4 Divide the arugula evenly among four bowls, and top each bowl with equal portions of salmon, asparagus, cabbage, cucumber, avocado, and nori pieces. Serve with the remaining dressing.

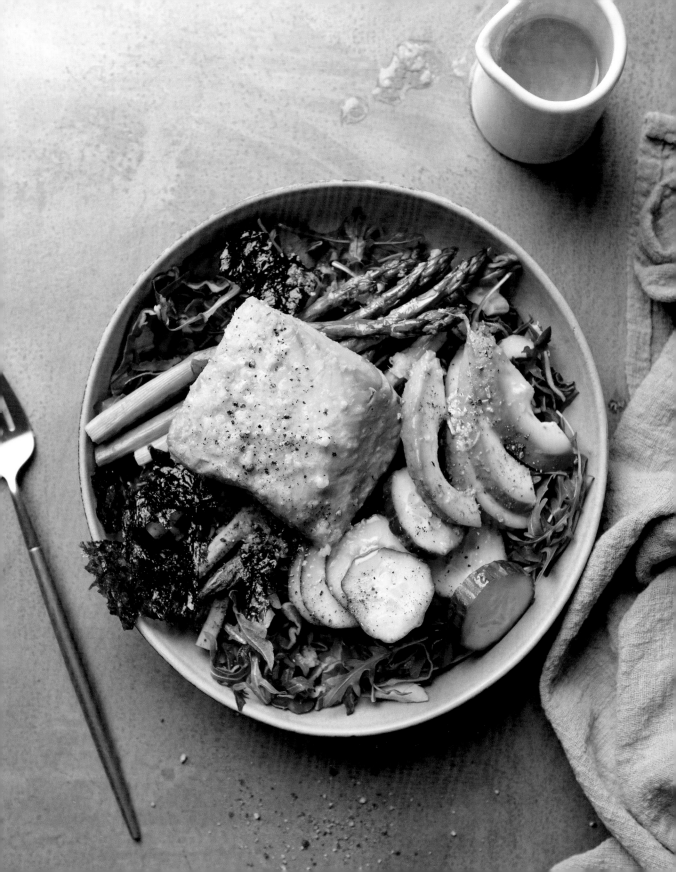

steamed sea bass
WITH CARROTS AND BOK CHOY

Cooking "en papillote," or sealed in a parchment paper pouch, is a delicious, easy, and healthy way to prepare fish. We particularly love this method because there's no need for extra oil and the cleanup is a cinch. Be sure to source wild-caught Chilean sea bass, or try black cod (sablefish) for an equally buttery option.

Yield **4 servings**	Prep Time **15 minutes, plus 1 hour to marinate**	Cook Time **20 minutes**	CLEANSE

2 tbsp chickpea miso

1 tbsp apple cider vinegar

½ tsp honey

Juice of 1 lime

3 carrots, cut into matchsticks

2 bunches baby bok choy, chopped (keep smaller leaves intact)

1 lb wild-caught Chilean sea bass, cut into 4 pieces (check for pinbones and remove with tweezers before cooking)

¼ cup sliced scallions (green and white parts), to garnish

Freshly ground black pepper, to serve

1 Preheat the oven to 375°F. Prepare four 15 x 15-inch pieces of parchment paper. Fold each piece of parchment in half.

2 In a small bowl, whisk together the chickpea miso, vinegar, honey, and lime juice.

3 Place a piece of parchment paper on a work surface. Just to the right of center, arrange about 8 carrot sticks and ½ cup bok choy. Place a piece of fish on top of the vegetables. Drizzle 1 tablespoon sauce over the fish.

4 To seal, fold the parchment paper over the top of the fish and veggies to cover completely. Starting at the bottom right corner, make small folds all the way around the edge to form a sealed packet. Place the packet on a rimmed baking sheet. Repeat to create packets for the remaining pieces of fish.

5 Place the baking sheet in the oven, and bake for 15 to 20 minutes. Remove from the oven and let rest for 5 minutes before opening the packets. When opening, be careful of hot steam. Garnish with scallions and black pepper just before serving.

note

Overfishing and the decline of our underwater ecosystem are two major concerns we all need to be aware of. When shopping for fish, look for wild-caught, certified sustainable seafood. Also, due to the ever-increasing toxins in our ocean waters, it's best to limit your seafood intake to just two to three times per week.

sweet miso black cod
WITH GARLICKY SPINACH

This is our version of the classic Japanese dish made famous by Chef Nobu Matsuhisa. Black cod, also called sablefish, is not actually a member of the cod family. Nonetheless, we love black cod because it's sustainably fished, full of omega-3s, and melt-in-your-mouth good!

Yield **2–4 servings**	Prep Time **20 minutes, plus 30 minutes to marinate**	Cook Time **15 minutes**	CLEANSE

2 tbsp coconut aminos

2 tbsp chickpea miso

2 tbsp rice vinegar

2 tsp raw honey

½ tsp toasted sesame oil

1 lb boneless black cod, cut into 2 pieces (check for pinbones and remove with tweezers before cooking)

½ tsp olive oil

1 clove garlic

1 bunch spinach, ends trimmed

Juice of ½ lemon (about 1 tbsp)

½ tsp black sesame seeds (optional), to garnish

1 In a medium bowl, whisk together the coconut aminos, miso, vinegar, honey, and sesame oil until smooth. Add the fish to the bowl, and spoon the marinade over top to coat all sides. Cover and refrigerate for 30 minutes.

2 Set the oven to broil. Place a lightly greased wire rack on a sheet pan, place the fish on the rack, skin side down (see tip), and spoon a little extra marinade on top of fish. Place under the broiler, and broil for 4 minutes.

3 Turn off the broiler and set the oven to 350°F. Let the fish bake for an additional 8 minutes or until the fish flakes easily with a fork.

4 Meanwhile, in a large nonstick skillet, heat the olive oil over medium-high heat. Add the garlic, cook for 1 minute, and add the spinach. Cook for 3 to 4 minutes, stirring occasionally or until wilted. Sprinkle with lemon juice, and remove from the heat.

5 Serve the spinach alongside the cod, garnished with sesame seeds, if using.

tip

If you don't have a rack that will fit on a baking sheet, you can line a baking sheet with foil and place the fish (skin side down) directly on the foil.

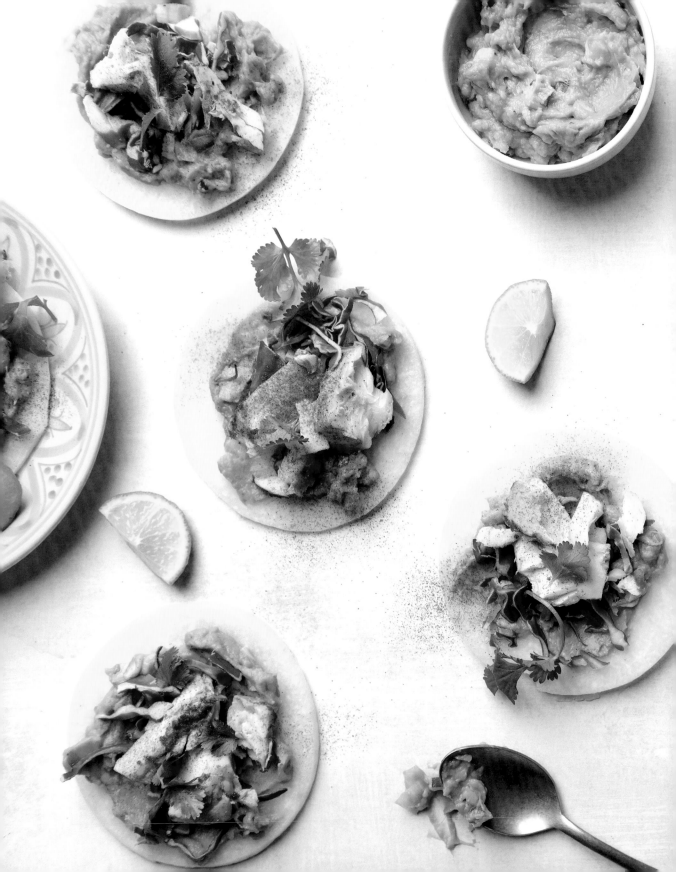

easy weeknight fish tacos

Jules made fish tacos in a skillet for years, but it always felt like such a production (not to mention the mess). This recipe fixes all that—and because the fish is baked, you don't have to stand over the hot stove the whole time. They're fresh, flavorful, and feature our favorite taco shell substitute—jicama!

Yield **2–3 servings**	Prep Time **15 minutes, plus 20 minutes to marinate**	Cook Time **15 minutes**	**LS** CLEANSE

1 lb halibut (or other whitefish), skin and bones removed

4–6 jicama tortillas (JicaTortillas brand recommended) or Bibb lettuce leaves

Simple Guacamole (page 184) or sliced avocado

½ cup finely shredded red cabbage

Fresh cilantro (optional), to garnish

For the marinade

2 tbsp olive oil

Juice and zest of 1 lime (about 1 tbsp each), plus lime wedges to serve

1 tsp ground cumin

1 tsp paprika

1 tsp chili powder

½ tsp Himalayan pink salt

1 To make the marinade, in a small bowl, whisk together all ingredients.

2 Place the fish in shallow glass baking dish, and pour the marinade over top, spreading to ensure the fish is fully coated. Place in the refrigerator to marinate for at least 20 minutes. Preheat the oven to 400°F.

3 Remove the fish from the refrigerator, and place in the oven. Bake for 15 minutes or until the fish flakes easily with a fork.

4 To assemble the tacos, place the jicama tortillas or lettuce leaves on a plate and top with guacamole or avocado, fish, and cabbage. Garnish with cilantro, if using, and lime wedges.

tip

To make your own jicama tortillas, wash and peel a large jicama. Cut in half crosswise, then cut into paper-thin slices with a sharp knife or the thinnest blade of a mandoline.

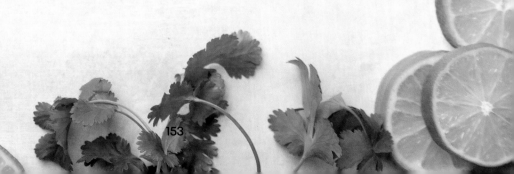

vegetables

millet vibrancy bowl 157

mexican rice bowl...158

curry rice salad 160

clean & simple stir-fry 161

celery toast 163

chipotle lime lentil burger 164

roasted cabbage 165

plant-powered not-meat balls.............................166

vegan chickpea curry...168

zucchini lasagna..169

quinoa flatbread pizza 171

mediterranean lettuce wrap 172

veggie sushi hand roll.. 173

fried cauliflower rice 174

sweet potato toast... 176

roasted rainbow veggies 177

how to build a vibrancy bowl

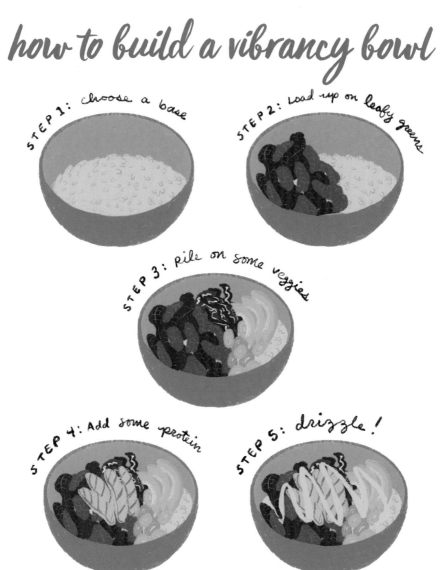

STEP 1: choose a base

STEP 2: Load up on leafy greens

STEP 3: pile on some veggies

STEP 4: Add some protein

STEP 5: drizzle!

The secret to a good vibrancy bowl is the drizzle, which ties all the flavors and textures together into a colorful, bountiful meal. Choose a gluten-free grain like quinoa or brown rice for the base, or use cauliflower or beet rice.

millet vibrancy bowl
WITH GREEN TAHINI DRESSING

Millet, one of our favorite gluten-free ancient grains, is technically a seed that packs a big nutritional punch. High in fiber, calcium, magnesium, and B vitamins, millet has a sweet but nutty flavor profile. This versatile vibrancy bowl is bursting with goodness and topped with a bright green tahini dressing—we love to sneak in more dark leafy greens and herbs wherever we can!

Yield **2 servings**	Prep Time **15 minutes**	Cook Time **35 minutes**	CLEANSE

1¾ cups water

1 cup uncooked millet, rinsed thoroughly with cold water and drained

2 cups **Roasted Rainbow Veggies** (page 177), warmed

2 tbsp dried wakame, soaked and drained (arame or another sea veggie would work, too)

½ cucumber, chopped

1 avocado, sliced

Kimchi, to garnish

Gomasio (see note), to garnish

For the dressing

⅓ cup raw tahini (Artisana Organics brand recommended)

½ cup water

1 small clove garlic, chopped

¼ cup freshly squeezed lemon juice

1 tsp apple cider vinegar

1 tsp honey

½ cup spinach, packed

¼ cup fresh Italian (flat-leaf) parsley, leaves and stems

1 tsp Himalayan pink salt

Freshly ground black pepper, to taste

1 In a small saucepan, bring the water to a boil. Add the millet, stir once, and cover. Reduce heat to low, and simmer for 20 minutes or until water is absorbed. Remove from heat and let the millet rest, covered, for 5 minutes. Fluff with a fork.

2 Meanwhile, make the dressing. In a high-speed blender, combine all ingredients and blend until smooth. If the dressing is too thick, add up to ¼ cup water to thin as needed. (Dressing can be refrigerated in an airtight container for up to 6 days.)

3 To assemble, divide the warm millet between two serving bowls. Arrange the warm roasted veggies, wakame, cucumber, and avocado on top. Top with desired amount of dressing, and garnish with kimchi and gomasio.

note
Gomasio is a traditional Japanese condiment consisting of sesame seeds and sea salt. Eden Foods makes a great organic option.

mexican rice bowl

We love Mexican food, and while we've been known to take down a bowl of tortilla chips with salsa, we wanted to create a corn- and dairy-free dish that was worthy of our 80:20 Plan. Easy to adapt for a family (serve with gluten-free tortillas) or meat lovers (just add shredded chicken), this comes together quickly on a weeknight. It also happens to be the dish that Jules loves to bring camping!

Yield **2 servings**	Prep Time **10 minutes , plus 4-hour soak**	Cook Time **5 minutes**	80:20

1 (15oz) can black beans, undrained

4 sprigs fresh cilantro

1 clove garlic, minced

Pinch of Himalayan pink salt

2 cups cooked brown rice

2 cups chopped romaine lettuce

½ cup sliced radishes

1 cup halved cherry tomatoes

1 avocado, sliced

For the dressing

1½ cups fresh cilantro

½ cup fresh Italian (flat-leaf) parsley

Juice and zest of 2 limes (about 1 tbsp zest)

3 cloves garlic, chopped

2 tsp honey

Himalayan pink salt, to taste

4 tbsp olive oil

For the cashew crema

¾ cup raw cashews, soaked for 4 hours and drained

1 tsp apple cider vinegar

2 tbsp freshly squeezed lemon juice

¾ tsp Himalayan pink salt

¼ cup water

1 In a small saucepan over low heat, combine the beans, cilantro, garlic, and salt. Simmer until all the liquid is absorbed. Set aside.

2 To make the dressing, in a high-speed blender, combine the cilantro, parsley, lime juice and zest, garlic, honey, and salt. Reduce blender to low and drizzle in the oil until well combined. Taste and add more salt if needed. (Dressing can be made ahead and refrigerated in an airtight glass container for up to 1 week.)

3 To make the cashew crema, in a food processor, combine the cashews, vinegar, lemon juice, salt, and water, and blend until smooth. (Crema can be made ahead and refrigerated in an airtight glass container for up to 1 week.)

4 To assemble the bowls, place even amounts of warm rice and lettuce in each bowl (about 1 cup each). Top with the warm beans, radishes, tomatoes, and avocado slices. Drizzle with dressing, and dollop cashew crema on top.

variation

You can swap cauliflower rice for the brown rice and/or add shredded chicken.

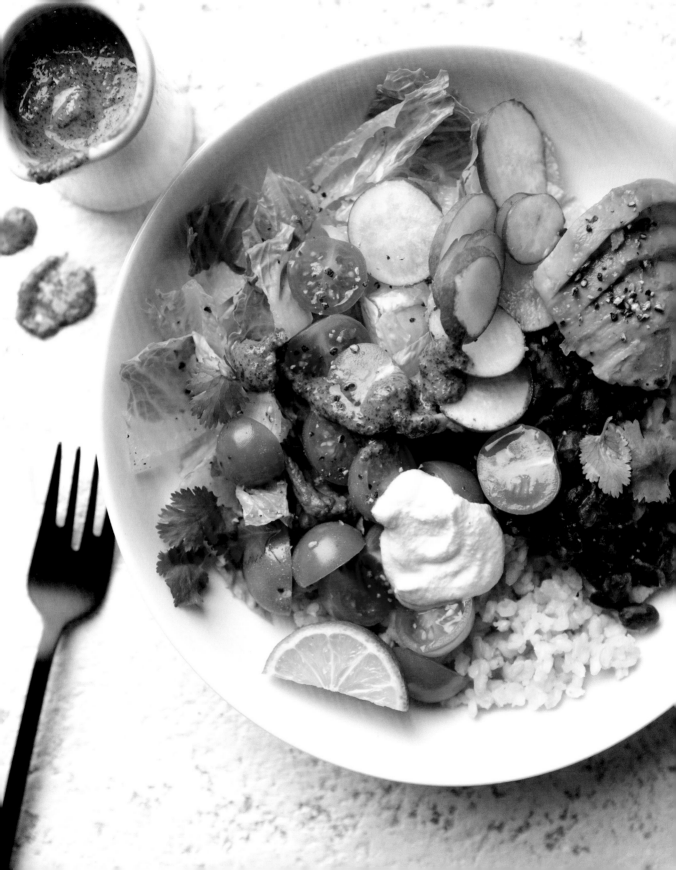

curry rice salad

Jo's mom has been serving this at block parties, potlucks, and family gatherings since Jo was a little kid, so we knew we had to feature this crowd-pleasing recipe. Curry, olives, and artichokes make this recipe super flavorful. The best part is that this dish is even better the second and third days.

Yield **8 servings**	Prep Time **15 minutes**	Cook Time **50 minutes**	CLEANSE

2 cups uncooked long-grain brown rice

1 tbsp + ½ tsp curry powder, divided

4 cups chicken broth

1 (14.5oz) can artichoke hearts, drained and quartered

½ cup sliced black olives

½ cup sliced green olives

4 scallions, chopped (white and light green parts only)

¾ tsp Himalayan pink salt

Freshly ground black pepper, to taste

2 tbsp olive oil

1 In a large pot, toast the rice for 3 to 5 minutes over high heat. Stir occasionally. Add 1 tablespoon curry powder and chicken broth, and stir. Cover and simmer for 45 minutes.

2 Transfer the cooked rice to a large bowl. Stir in the artichokes, black and green olives, and scallions. Add the salt, pepper, oil, and remaining ½ teaspoon curry powder. Serve warm or chill in the refrigerator for a refreshing cold salad.

clean & simple stir-fry

This super-simple stir-fry is one of our staples during the cleanse. Warm, nutrient-dense, and filled with color and texture, it shows how delicious simple food can be. Use this recipe as a guide and add your favorite vegetables and herbs; just be sure they are fresh, organic, and in season, when possible.

Yield **2 servings**	Prep Time **15 minutes**	Cook Time **10 minutes**	**LS** CLEANSE

¾ cup vegetable broth or water, divided

2 cloves garlic, minced

1 tbsp minced fresh ginger

1 cup julienned carrots

1 cup broccoli florets

1 cup cauliflower florets

1 cup sliced shiitake mushrooms

1 cup sugar snap pea or snow peas

To serve

Cooked cauliflower rice, zucchini noodles, or steamed kale (optional)

¼ cup chopped fresh cilantro

¼ cup chopped fresh basil

½ cup mung beans

Coconut aminos or ume plum vinegar, to taste

1 In a large sauté pan, heat 4 tablespoons vegetable broth over medium-high heat. When the broth starts to steam, add the garlic and ginger. Sauté for about 1 minute or until fragrant.

2 Add the carrots and cook for 2 to 3 minutes. Add more broth, 1 tablespoon at a time, as needed. Add the broccoli, cauliflower, and mushrooms, and cook for another 4 to 5 minutes. Add the snap peas and cook for another 2 to 3 minutes or until they are bright green but still crisp.

3 Serve over cauliflower rice, zucchini noodles, or steamed kale, if using. Top with cilantro, basil, and mung beans. Season with coconut aminos or ume plum vinegar to taste.

note

This is a great recipe for Purification, minus the coconut aminos and ume plum vinegar.

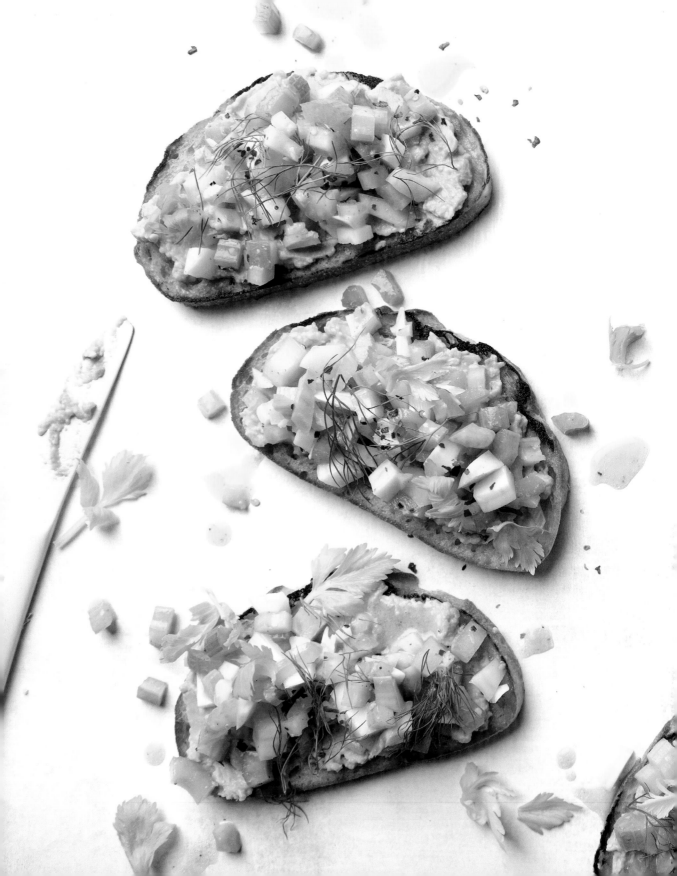

celery toast

Move over avocado toast, there's a new kid in town! Celery toast takes what we love about avocado toast—a thick layer of smashed avocado—and adds epic texture and crunch. Look out, because you're gonna want to soak up the lemony-garlic marinade with an extra piece of crusty, gluten-free bread.

Yield **4 servings**	Prep Time **15 minutes**	Cook Time **None**	80:20

¼ cup olive oil

Juice of ½ lemon

1 large clove garlic, finely minced

2 tsp brown mustard

Pinch of Himalayan pink salt

Freshly ground black pepper, to taste

1½ cups finely chopped celery (about 3 large stalks)

½ cup finely chopped fennel (about ⅓ bulb fennel), fronds reserved for garnish

4 slices crusty, gluten-free bread, toasted

1 avocado, mashed

Red pepper flakes, to taste

1 In a medium bowl, whisk together the oil, lemon juice, garlic, mustard, salt, and pepper. Add the celery and fennel, and toss to combine.

2 Top each piece of toasted bread with a layer of mashed avocado. Pile about ¼ cup celery-fennel mixture on each piece, and sprinkle with red pepper flakes.

3 Leftover celery-fennel mixture can be refrigerated in an airtight glass container for up to 1 week.

variation

The celery-fennel mixture makes a great topper or addition to any salad. We especially love it over arugula, topped with avocado.

chipotle lime lentil burgers

On a quest to make a plant-based burger that didn't fall apart or taste dry and boring, the Chipotle Lime Lentil Burger was born. Bursting with flavor, these lentil burgers are loaded with veggies and spices. The flaxseeds help bind them together, so they're chewy and won't fall apart when cooked.

Yield **6 burgers**	Prep Time **30 minutes**	Cook Time **65 minutes**	CLEANSE

1 cup uncooked green lentils

½ cup finely chopped sweet yellow onion

2 cloves garlic, minced

1 cup chopped portobello mushrooms

1 cup shredded carrots

½ tbsp olive oil

2 tbsp coconut aminos

½ cup ground flaxseeds

½ tsp ground cumin

½ tsp ground coriander

½ tsp paprika

¼ tsp chipotle powder

Juice and zest of 1 lime

½ tsp Himalayan pink salt

½ tsp freshly ground black pepper

To serve (optional)
Mixed greens or lettuce leaves

Egg-Free Avocado Mayo
  (page 245)

Sprouts

Sliced avocado

1 Place the lentils in a large stock pot, and add water to cover (3–4 cups). Bring to a boil. Reduce the heat and simmer for 20 minutes or until the lentils are tender. Drain and set aside.

2 Meanwhile, preheat the oven to 400°F. In a large bowl, combine the onion, garlic, mushrooms, and carrots. Add the oil, and toss to coat vegetables. Spread the vegetables on a baking sheet lined with parchment paper. Place in the oven for 15 minutes or until vegetables are tender.

3 In a food processor, combine the lentils, roasted vegetables, coconut aminos, ground flaxseeds, cumin, coriander, paprika, chipotle, lime juice and zest, salt, and pepper. Pulse until the mixture is smooth but still has texture. Be careful not to overmix.

4 Line a separate baking sheet with parchment paper, and reduce the oven temperature to 350°F. Form the mixture into 6 patties. Place on the prepared baking sheet, and bake for 30 minutes, flipping the patties once halfway through. Enjoy over mixed greens or serve on a butter lettuce "bun" topped with avocado mayo, sprouts, and avocado, if using.

roasted cabbage

Cabbage has to be the most underrated vegetable of all time. Loaded with antioxidants and anti-inflammatory properties, it's been shown to play a crucial part in fighting chronic disease and building a healthy gut microbiome. This recipe is delicious with salmon or salad greens.

Yield **4 servings**	Prep Time **15 minutes**	Cook Time **45 minutes**	CLEANSE

2 heads green cabbage, chopped

3 carrots, roughly chopped

2 tbsp coconut or olive oil

½ tsp Himalayan pink salt

Freshly ground black pepper, to taste

2 cloves garlic, minced

2–3 scallions (green and white parts), sliced, to garnish

Handful of fresh cilantro, to garnish

For the dressing

2 tbsp apple cider vinegar

2 tbsp sesame oil

2 tbsp coconut aminos

1 tbsp grated fresh ginger

¼ tsp red pepper flakes

1 Position a rack in the center of the oven, and preheat to 425°F. Line a baking sheet with parchment paper.

2 On the prepared baking sheet, toss the cabbage and carrots with the coconut oil, salt, and a few grinds of pepper. Spread the cabbage evenly on the baking sheet (it's okay if the cabbage is crowded; it will shrink as it roasts), and roast, tossing every 10 minutes, for 35 to 45 minutes or until the cabbage is tender and golden brown. In the last 5 minutes of cooking, add the garlic.

3 To make the dressing, in a small bowl, whisk together all ingredients.

4 Transfer the cabbage to a large bowl, and toss with 2 tablespoons dressing. Season to taste with additional dressing, and garnish with scallions and cilantro.

plant-powered not-meat balls
WITH ZOODLES AND NO–MATO MARINARA

Most store-bought meatballs—vegan or not—are loaded with fillers and other questionable ingredients. Our simple, 10-ingredient, plant-based meatballs are full of flavor, packed with veggies, won't fall apart, and are bean-free. The perfect "meat" ball, if you ask us! Serve atop a bed of zucchini noodles along with our No-Mato Marinara for a clean, vegan twist on classic spaghetti and meatballs.

Yield **16 balls**	Prep Time **20 minutes**	Cook Time **45 minutes**	80:20

2 tbsp olive oil

1 yellow onion, finely chopped

10 oz cremini mushrooms, chopped

2 cloves garlic, chopped

1½ cups cooked quinoa, cold or
  room temperature

½ cup almond flour

2 tsp dried Italian seasoning

¼ tsp red pepper flakes

1 tsp Himalayan pink salt

Freshly ground black pepper,
  to taste

To serve

Cooked spiralized zucchini or
  spaghetti squash

No-Mato Marinara (page 244)

Fresh basil

1 In a large skillet, heat the oil over medium-high heat. Add the onion and sauté for about 7 minutes or until fragrant. Add the mushrooms, increase the heat to medium-high, and cook for 10 to 15 minutes. (Wait until the liquid evaporates, and keep cooking the mushrooms until they brown nicely.) Add the garlic, stir, and transfer the mixture to a large bowl. Let cool to room temperature.

2 While the mushroom mixture cools, preheat the oven to 350°F and line a rimmed baking sheet with parchment paper.

3 In a food processor, combine the cooled mushroom mixture and the cooked quinoa. Blend well until a hearty mixture is formed. (It should stick together.) Return the mixture to the large bowl, and add the almond flour, Italian seasoning, red pepper flakes, salt, and pepper. Stir to combine.

4 Using a heaping tablespoon (about 2 tablespoons per ball) of mixture, form balls using damp hands. Place them on the prepared baking sheet, and bake for 30 minutes, turning halfway through.

5 Serve warm over spiralized zucchini or roasted spaghetti squash, and top with No-Mato Marinara and fresh basil.

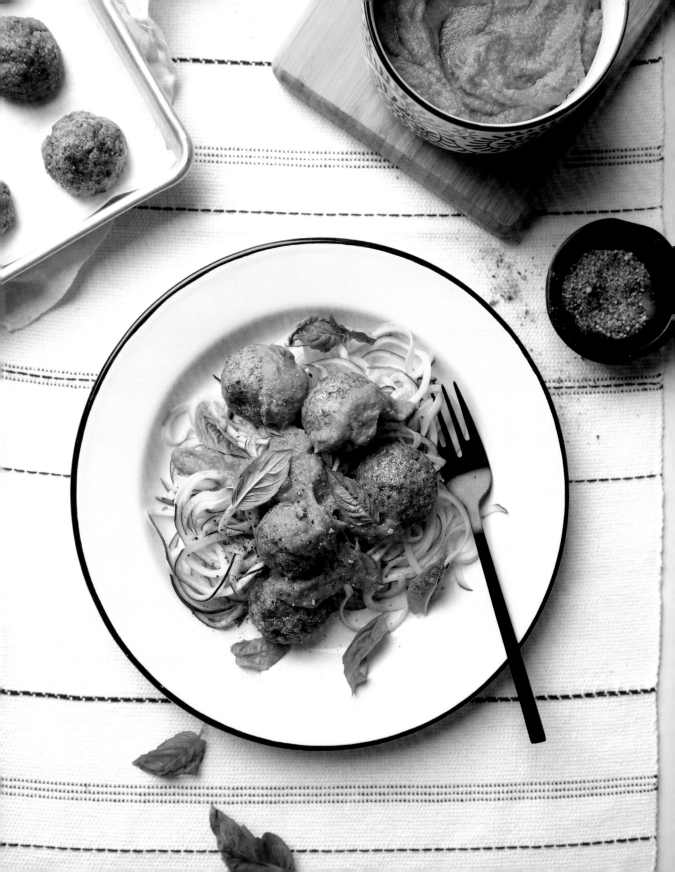

vegan chickpea curry

If you're looking for warm, nourishing comfort food, look no further. This mild vegan curry is super easy to whip together any night of the week, using mostly simple pantry items. It's a one-pot meal that's both cleanse friendly and a family favorite.

Yield **4 servings**	Prep Time **10 minutes**	Cook Time **20 minutes**	CLEANSE

1 tsp coconut oil

1 yellow onion, diced

2 cloves garlic, minced

1 tbsp minced fresh ginger

2 carrots, diced

1 tbsp curry powder

2 cups cooked or canned
  chickpeas, drained

1 (13.5oz) can full-fat coconut milk

Juice of ½ lime

Himalayan pink salt and freshly
  ground black pepper, to taste

Fresh cilantro or scallions, chopped
  (optional), to garnish

1 head curly kale, stems removed,
  chopped and steamed, or
  4–8 cups cooked cauliflower rice

1 In a Dutch oven or large skillet, melt the oil over medium-high heat. Add the onion, and sauté for 5 minutes.

2 Add the garlic, ginger, carrots, and curry powder. Cook, stirring frequently, until the carrots start to soften. Stir in the chickpeas and coconut milk. Bring to a boil and then reduce heat to medium-low. Simmer curry for about 10 minutes or until slightly reduced.

3 Stir in the lime juice. Taste and season with salt and pepper. Garnish with fresh cilantro or scallions, if using. Serve hot over steamed kale or cauliflower rice.

zucchini lasagna
WITH RICOTTA "CHEESE"

This veggie lasagna checks all the boxes: cleanse-approved, dairy-free, gluten-free, nightshade-free, veggie-packed, and nutrient-dense. It's the epitome of comfort food—without the gas, bloat, or food coma—and pairs delightfully with a simple green salad or our Spicy Kale Caesar.

Yield **6 servings**	Prep Time **5 minutes, plus 4-hour soak**	Cook Time **55 minutes**	**LS** CLEANSE

2 summer squash, very thinly sliced lengthwise

3 zucchini, very thinly sliced lengthwise

2 bulbs fennel, very thinly sliced

¼ cup olive oil

1 tsp Himalayan pink salt

2 cups **No-Mato Marinara** (page 244)

2 cups baby spinach, packed

For the ricotta "cheese"

1 cup raw cashews, soaked for 4 hours and drained

2 tbsp olive oil

Juice of 1 lemon

1 tsp Himalayan pink salt

¼ cup water

1 tsp dried oregano

Pinch of freshly ground black pepper

1 Preheat the oven to 400°F and line two baking sheets with parchment paper. In a large bowl, toss the summer squash, zucchini, and fennel with the oil and salt. Spread the vegetables in a single layer on the prepared baking sheets, and roast for 20 to 25 minutes or until they start to brown and caramelize around the edges. Remove from the oven and set aside to cool. Reduce the oven temperature to 350°F.

2 To make the ricotta "cheese," in a food processor, combine the cashews, oil, lemon juice, salt, and water. Process until a smooth paste forms. (You may need to add a bit more water.) Transfer the mixture to a medium bowl, and whisk in the oregano and pepper.

3 Spread about ½ cup marinara sauce on the bottom of a 9 x 9-inch glass baking dish. Cover the sauce with a layer of zucchini and summer squash. Next, layer some of the roasted fennel and top with dollops of ricotta "cheese." Spread a layer of spinach leaves on top. Spoon about ½ cup marinara sauce over the spinach, covering the entire layer.

4 Continue to layer the remaining zucchini, summer squash, fennel, ricotta "cheese," spinach, and No-Mato Sauce until the top of the dish is reached (to make about 3 layers). Reserve some ricotta "cheese" to dollop on the very top of the dish.

5 Bake for 30 minutes. Allow to cool for 5 minutes before serving.

 tips

A mandoline is helpful when cutting thin slices of squash, zucchini, and fennel (although not required).

When not cleansing, simplify this recipe by using a store-bought sugar-free marinara sauce.

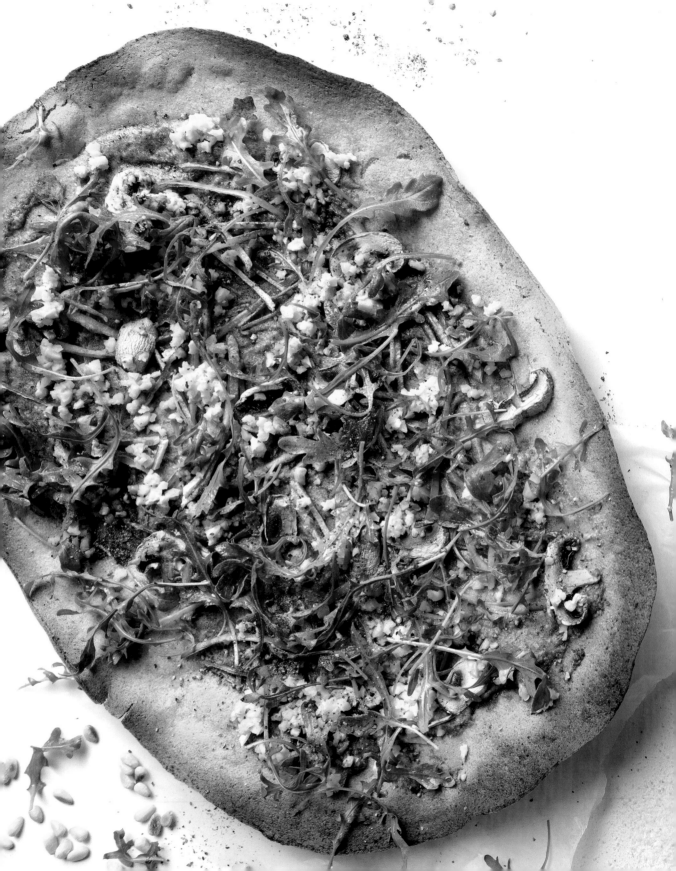

quinoa flatbread pizza
WITH ARUGULA PESTO

Healthy, guilt-free pizza? Yes, please! If the thought of making your own flatbread seems intimidating, do not worry. This quinoa crust comes together surprisingly easily. Topped with fresh pesto and loaded with spicy arugula, one of our favorite dark leafy greens, this one is sure to be a crowd pleaser.

| Yield **1 pizza** | Prep Time **20 minutes, plus overnight soak** | Cook Time **35 minutes** | CLEANSE |

For the crust

¾ cup uncooked quinoa, soaked overnight, rinsed, and drained

¾ cup uncooked millet, soaked overnight, rinsed, and drained

½ cup water

1 tbsp olive oil

½ tsp Himalayan pink salt

¼ cup fresh basil, lightly packed

Toppings

¾ cup **Arugula Pesto** (page 247)

¼ red onion, thinly sliced

¼ cup sliced cremini mushrooms

¼ cup **Cashew Feta** (optional, page 243; skip when cleansing)

1 tbsp balsamic vinegar

1 cup baby arugula

1 tsp olive oil

Himalayan pink salt and freshly ground black pepper, to taste

1 Preheat the oven to 450°F. Line a baking sheet with parchment paper.

2 In a food processor, combine the quinoa, millet, water, oil, and salt. Blend until you get a thick, pancake batter–like consistency. Add the basil and another 3 tablespoons water to thin (if needed). Pour the batter onto the prepared baking sheet, spreading it out evenly with a spatula.

3 Place in the oven, and bake for 15 minutes. Remove from the oven, carefully flip the crust, and return to the oven to bake for 6 to 8 minutes more. Remove from the oven and allow to cool slightly.

4 When cool enough to handle, spread the pesto over the flatbread. Top with onions, mushrooms, and cashew feta, if using. Drizzle with balsamic vinegar, and return to the oven for 5 to 10 minutes.

5 Toss the arugula in the oil, salt, and pepper. Add to top of pizza. Cut and serve immediately.

tip

The sky's the limit in the topping department! Jules loves zucchini, tomatoes, mushrooms, and feta (when not cleansing).

mediterranean lettuce wrap

Packed with savory flavors, this plant-powered lettuce wrap is our new favorite lunch—and it's kid friendly, too! It packs well and is easy to eat. The star ingredient is our Roasted Garlic Cauliflower Hummus, which is seriously the best bean-free hummus we've ever had (if we do say so ourselves)!

Yield **1 wrap**	Prep Time **15 minutes**	Cook Time **None**	CLEANSE

6 large romaine lettuce leaves, thick ribs trimmed

¼ cup **Roasted Garlic Cauliflower Hummus** (page 181)

¼ cup baby spinach, finely chopped

¼ English cucumber, sliced (about 8 slices)

⅓ red onion, thinly sliced

½ avocado, sliced

¼ cup Kalamata olives

½ cup **Cashew Feta** (page 243)

1 To make the wrap, place a piece of parchment paper on a cutting board or work surface. Layer romaine leaves horizontally in the center of the parchment paper to create a lettuce base about 8 to 9 inches wide.

2 Fill the wrap by spreading the garlic cauliflower hummus in the center of the romaine leaves. Layer on the spinach, cucumber, onion, avocado, olives, and cashew feta.

3 When you have all your fillings in place, starting at the end closest to you, roll the lettuce wraps burrito-style, as tightly as possible, using the parchment paper as your base. Halfway through rolling, tuck the ends of the wrap toward the center and then continue to roll the lettuce wrap, keeping the parchment paper as taut as possible.

4 Cut the wrap in half, wrap in another piece of parchment paper, and refrigerate until ready to eat.

note

Creating a romaine wrap in parchment paper is not as hard as it sounds. Think deli-style wrap or rolling a burrito. With practice, you'll get the hang of this and be so glad you did. These wraps are the perfect to-go lunch, and the filling combinations are endless.

veggie sushi hand roll

A sushi hand roll may look and sound gourmet, but this veggie roll is a quick and easy lunch. It's also easily customized, so feel free to substitute whatever fresh veggies you have on hand—pun intended!

Yield **2 servings**	Prep Time **15 minutes**	Cook Time **None**	CLEANSE

1 avocado

Squeeze of lemon or lime juice

Dash of Himalayan pink salt

2 nori sheets, cut in half

⅓ English cucumber, cut into matchsticks

1 carrot, cut in matchsticks

1 daikon, cut into matchsticks

1 cup shredded red cabbage

2 scallions, trimmed and sliced in half lengthwise

Handful of your favorite sprouts

¼ cup gomasio (Eden Foods brand recommended)

½ cup coconut aminos, to serve

Sugar-free sriracha sauce (optional; Picaflor brand recommeded), to serve

1   In a small bowl, mash the avocado with the lemon or lime juice and salt.

2   Place the nori sheets on a flat work surface, shiny sides down. Evenly divide the cucumber, carrots, daikon, cabbage, avocado, scallions, and sprouts among the nori sheets; sprinkle with gomasio; and roll. To seal the rolls, run a wet paper towel across the inside edge of the nori.

3   Serve with coconut aminos for dipping and a splash of sugar-free Sriracha, if using.

fried cauliflower rice

Cauliflower rice has made its debut on the health food scene in a major way in the last few years. You can even find it already "riced" in the frozen section of many grocery stores. Although we prefer using fresh cauliflower when possible, this is still an easy weeknight dinner that utilizes ingredients we often have on hand. Plus, it's grain-free and a major upgrade to any Chinese takeout.

Yield **4 servings**	Prep Time **10 minutes**	Cook Time **15 minutes**	80:20

1½ tbsp olive oil, divided

Pinch of Himalayan pink salt

Pinch of freshly ground black pepper

2 eggs, beaten

1 small head cauliflower, cut into florets

1 medium onion, diced

2 tbsp grated fresh ginger

1 large clove garlic, minced

1 cup sliced cremini mushrooms

2 carrots, finely diced

2 tbsp coconut aminos

1 tbsp rice wine vinegar

½ cup frozen peas

Chopped fresh cilantro, to garnish

3 scallions, sliced, to garnish

1 In a small nonstick skillet, heat ½ tablespoon oil over medium heat. Add the salt and pepper to the beaten eggs and pour into the skillet. Cook for 1 to 2 minutes or until the bottom of the egg has set. Using a spatula, fold over the egg to make an omelet. Remove from heat and set aside.

2 In a food processor, pulse the cauliflower until it has a fine, rice-like texture. Set aside.

3 In a large skillet, warm the remaining 1 tablespoon oil over medium-high heat. Add the onion, ginger, and garlic, and sauté for 3 to 4 minutes or until translucent. Add the mushrooms and carrots, and sauté for about 5 minutes or until the mushrooms are golden and the carrots are tender.

4 Add the cauliflower rice and cook, covered, stirring occasionally, for 5 to 8 minutes or until tender. Stir in the coconut aminos and rice wine vinegar. Add the frozen peas, and stir until thawed and heated through.

5 Meanwhile, roll and slice the omelet into ribbons. Add to the skillet and give a quick stir to warm. Garnish with cilantro and scallions just before serving.

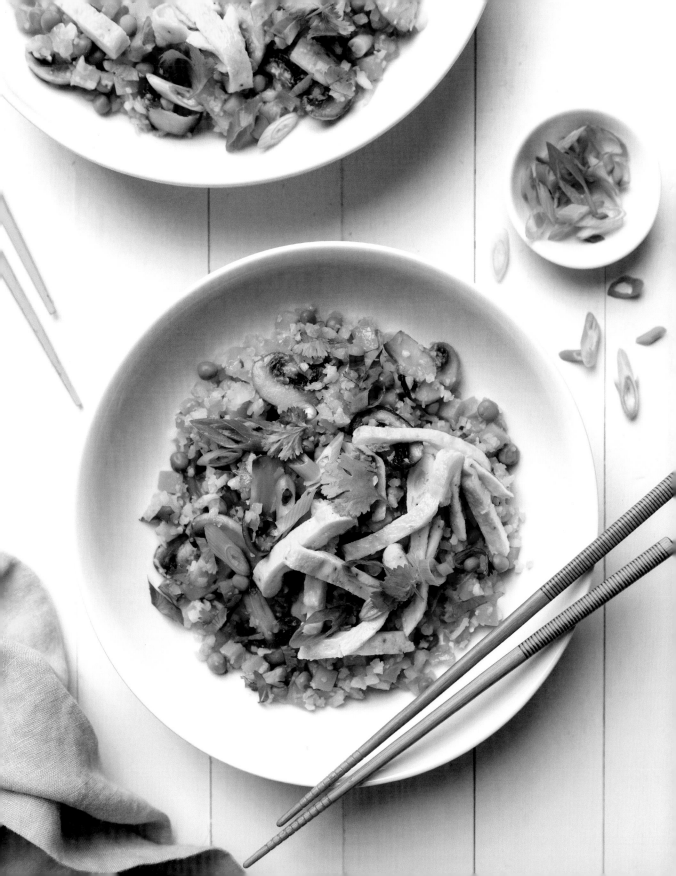

sweet potato toast

We're always looking for ways to incorporate more veggies in place of "filler" foods, like bread. Enter, sweet potatoes! When thinly sliced and par baked, they make the perfect carrier for all the toppings we love.

Yield **5 slices**	Prep Time **5 minutes**	Cook Time **20 minutes**	CLEANSE

1 large sweet potato, washed and dried

Toppings of choice

1 Preheat the oven to 350°F. Trim both ends of the sweet potato. Slice the sweet potato lengthwise into ¼-inch slices. (Depending on the size of your sweet potato, you should have about 5 slices.) Arrange the slices in a single layer on a wire rack or a baking sheet lined with parchment paper.

2 Bake for 15 to 20 minutes or until the potatoes are tender but not fully cooked. Keep an eye on them so they don't burn. Remove from the oven, and allow the slices to cool before transferring them to an airtight container. Store in the refrigerator for up to 4 days.

3 When ready to eat, place the sweet potato slices in a toaster oven. Toast until the edges are crispy, and add toppings as desired.

Avocado Lime

½ avocado

Juice of ½ lime

Himalayan pink salt, to taste

In a small bowl, mash the avocado with the lime juice. Spread the mashed avocado onto the toasted sweet potato slices, and sprinkle with salt.

Almond Butter (80:20)

2 tbsp raw almond butter

1 banana, sliced

Dash of ground cinnamon

Spread almond butter onto the toasted sweet potato slices. Top with sliced banana and a sprinkle of cinnamon.

Beet Hummus

2 tbsp **Beet Hummus** (page 182)

Handful of arugula

Juice of ½ lemon

Himalayan pink salt, to taste

Spread the beet hummus onto the toasted sweet potato slices. Top with a handful of fresh arugula, a squeeze of lemon juice, and a sprinkle of salt.

roasted rainbow veggies

"Eat the rainbow" is a fun and simple way to remember to eat a variety of fruits and vegetables in order to get all the vitamins and minerals you need for vibrant health. Have fun mixing up this recipe with your veggies of choice—the only rule is to keep it colorful! And don't forget to use fresh herbs whenever possible. They really enhance the flavor and benefits of this dish.

Yield **8 servings**	Prep Time **20 minutes**	Cook Time **45 minutes**	CLEANSE

8 rainbow carrots, scrubbed and halved lengthwise

2 small beets, trimmed, peeled, and quartered

2 cups (about 8oz) halved Brussels sprouts

4 tbsp olive oil, divided

2 tsp Himalayan pink salt, divided

½ tsp freshly ground black pepper, divided

1–2 tbsp chopped fresh herbs such as thyme, rosemary, or oregano (optional), divided

2 bulbs fennel, thinly sliced

1 head broccoli, cut into florets

1 head cauliflower, cut into florets

1 Preheat the oven to 425°F. Line two baking sheets with parchment paper or silicone liners.

2 On one baking sheet, toss the carrots, beets, and Brussels sprouts with 2 tablespoons oil, 1 teaspoon salt, ¼ teaspoon pepper, and half of the herbs, if using. Spread evenly over the sheet.

3 On the other baking sheet, toss the fennel, broccoli, and cauliflower with the remaining 2 tablespoons oil, 1 teaspoon salt, ¼ teaspoon pepper, and herbs (if using). Spread evenly over the sheet.

4 Place both baking sheets in the oven, and roast for about 25 minutes, tossing at the halfway point. The carrots, beets, and Brussels sprouts may need an additional 10 to 15 minutes. When the veggies are fork-tender, remove from the oven and season with additional salt and pepper, to taste. Leftovers can be refrigerated in an airtight glass container for up to 4 days.

variation

For oil-free roasted veggies, steam the carrots, beets, and Brussels sprouts on the stove in a steamer basket until fork-tender, then transfer to a sheet pan for roasting. Broccoli and cauliflower can be placed on a baking sheet lined with parchment paper and roasted without oil.

dips, snacks & starters

garlicky dill dip...180

roasted garlic cauliflower hummus 181

beet hummus 182

simple guacamole 184

plant-powered queso dip..185

chickpea rosemary flatbread 187

spinach artichoke dip...188

garlic yam spread 189

superfood bars.. 190

golden flaxseed crackers...192

super seaweed crackers 193

curry roasted cashews 195

roasted chickpeas 196

parsnip fries 197

sesame cauli wings..198

garlicky dill dip

We love a good dip and always have one on hand during cleanse time. This is great for a filling snack with raw veggies or our Parsnip Fries. Loaded with flavor, fresh dill is a must in this recipe!

| Yield **1 cup** | Prep Time **10 minutes, plus 1-hour soak** | Cook Time **None** | CLEANSE |

1 cup raw pumpkin seeds, soaked in warm water for 1 hour and drained

¾ tsp Himalayan pink salt

3 cloves garlic

½ cup fresh dill (including some stems)

¼ cup freshly squeezed lemon juice

½ cup olive oil

¼ cup water

1. In a food processor, blend the pumpkin seeds for about 1 minute or until smooth.

2. Add the salt, garlic, dill, lemon juice, and oil. Blend for 5 minutes or until smooth and creamy, scraping the sides as necessary. Slowly add the water, 1 tablespoon at a time, until desired consistency is reached.

roasted garlic cauliflower hummus

This no-bean hummus was inspired by our Zucchini Hummus, one of Jules' favorite recipes from our first book. This time around, we roasted the cauliflower and the garlic, giving us a delicious and earthy dip. It's perfect for a quick snack with crudité or smeared in a wrap.

Yield **2 cups**	Prep Time **15 minutes**	Cook Time **35 minutes**	**LS** CLEANSE

5–6 cups cauliflower florets

4½ tbsp olive oil, divided

Pinch + 1 tsp Himalayan pink salt, divided

1 head garlic, papery outer layers removed

3 tbsp freshly squeezed lemon juice

2 tbsp raw tahini (Artisana Organics brand recommended)

¼ tsp ground cumin

2 tbsp cold water

¼ tsp freshly ground black pepper

Sliced carrots, celery, and cucumber (optional), to serve

1. Preheat the oven to 400°F. Line a baking sheet with parchment paper.

2. In a large bowl, toss the cauliflower with 2 tablespoons oil to coat. Spread the cauliflower evenly on the prepared baking sheet, and sprinkle with a pinch of salt. Set aside.

3. Slice ¼ to ½ inch from the top of the garlic head, exposing the individual cloves (pointy side). Place the garlic head (cut side up) on a piece of foil, drizzle with ½ tablespoon oil, using your fingers to rub the oil into the exposed cloves. Seal the foil around the head of garlic completely.

4. Place the foil-wrapped garlic on the baking sheet (cut side up) with the cauliflower. Place in the oven, and roast for 35 minutes, turning the cauliflower at the halfway mark. Remove from the oven, unwrap the garlic, and set aside to cool. When the garlic is cool to touch, squeeze out 6 cloves (see note).

5. In a food processor, combine the 6 roasted garlic cloves, lemon juice, tahini, cumin, and remaining 1 teaspoon salt. Process for 1 minute or until smooth, stopping to scrape down the sides as necessary. With the motor running, drizzle in the cold water and then the remaining 2 tablespoons oil. Finally, add the roasted cauliflower and process for 2 minutes or until the mixture is smooth and creamy. Taste and season with pepper.

6. Serve immediately (or chill for 20 minutes) with carrots, celery, and cucumber slices, if using. Store in an airtight container in the refrigerator for up to 3 days.

 tip

The remaining roasted garlic can be used as a spread on Golden Flaxseed Crackers (page 192) or blended in a salad dressing.

beet hummus

This vibrant hummus is a favorite from our first book. Made with roasted beets, it is as beautiful in its hot pink appearance as it is flavorful and nutritious. High in fiber, antioxidants, calcium, iron, and protein, this colorful and creamy hummus is a must for your next gathering.

Yield **1½ cups**	Prep Time **15 minutes**	Cook Time **20 minutes**	CLEANSE

3 medium beets, peeled and quartered

3 tbsp olive oil, divided

2 tbsp raw tahini (Artisana Organics brand recommended)

¼ cup freshly squeezed lemon juice

1 clove garlic, minced

½ tsp Himalayan pink salt

½ tsp freshly ground black pepper

Sliced cucumber (optional), to serve

Sliced carrots (optional), to serve

Super Seaweed Crackers (optional, page 193), to serve

1   Preheat the oven to 375° F. Place the beets in a glass baking dish, and toss to coat with 1 tablespoon oil. Cover with foil and bake for 20 minutes or until the beets are soft.

2   In a food processor, process the cooked beets, tahini, lemon juice, garlic, remaining 2 tablespoons oil, salt, and pepper until smooth.

3   Cover and refrigerate for at least 1 hour to allow flavors to develop. Serve with sliced cucumbers, carrots, and seaweed crackers, if using. Refrigerate leftovers in an airtight container for up to 1 week.

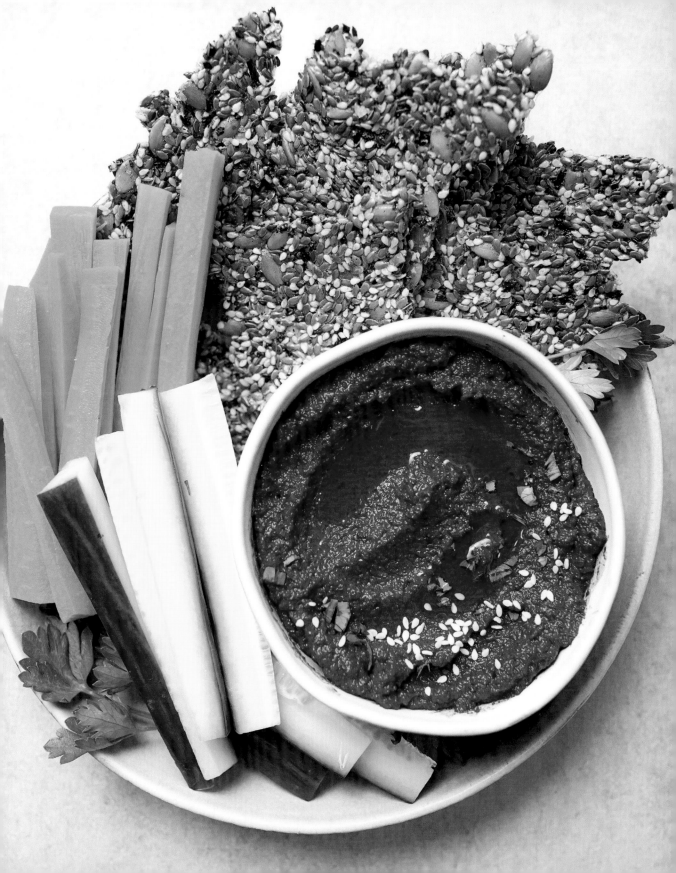

simple guacamole

This quick and easy guac is a staple in Jules' household. Serve it with our Mexican Rice Bowl, Easy Weeknight Fish Tacos, or just scoop it up with some veggie sticks for a filling snack.

Yield **1½ cups**	Prep Time **10 minutes**	Cook Time **None**	CLEANSE

2 ripe avocados, halved and pitted

Juice of ½ lime

1 clove garlic, finely minced

¼ cup chopped red onion

2 tbsp finely chopped fresh cilantro

½ tsp Himalayan pink salt

Freshly ground black pepper, to taste

1 Scoop out avocado flesh and place in a bowl. Using a fork, roughly mash the avocado.

2 Add the lime juice, garlic, onion, and cilantro. Season with salt and pepper, and stir to combine. Serve immediately to avoid browning.

plant-powered queso dip

Your guests will never guess the magical secret ingredient in this vegan queso dip! Butternut squash gives this dip a beautiful cheese-like hue. With chili powder, smoked paprika, and nutritional yeast adding loads of flavor, all we can say is, "Yum!" Serve this warm with crudité or grain-free chips, such as Siete brand.

Yield **8–10 servings**	Prep Time **10 minutes, plus 1-hour soak**	Cook Time **15 minutes**	80:20

1 (14.5oz) can butternut squash

½ cup roughly chopped yellow onion

½ cup raw cashews, soaked for 1 hour and drained

½ cup water

1 (14.5oz) can diced tomatoes

1½ tsp ground cumin

1 tsp chili powder

½–1 tsp smoked paprika

½ cup nutritional yeast

2 cloves garlic, minced

1 jalapeño, diced

3 tbsp freshly squeezed lime juice

¼ tsp Himalayan pink salt

1 In a high-speed blender, combine the squash, onion, cashews, and water. Blend until smooth.

2 Transfer the mixture to a medium saucepan, and place over medium heat. Add the tomatoes, cumin, chili powder, ½ teaspoon smoked paprika, nutritional yeast, garlic, jalapeño, lime juice, and salt, and mix well. Cook, stirring frequently, for about 15 minutes to let flavors develop. Taste and adjust smoked paprika to your liking.

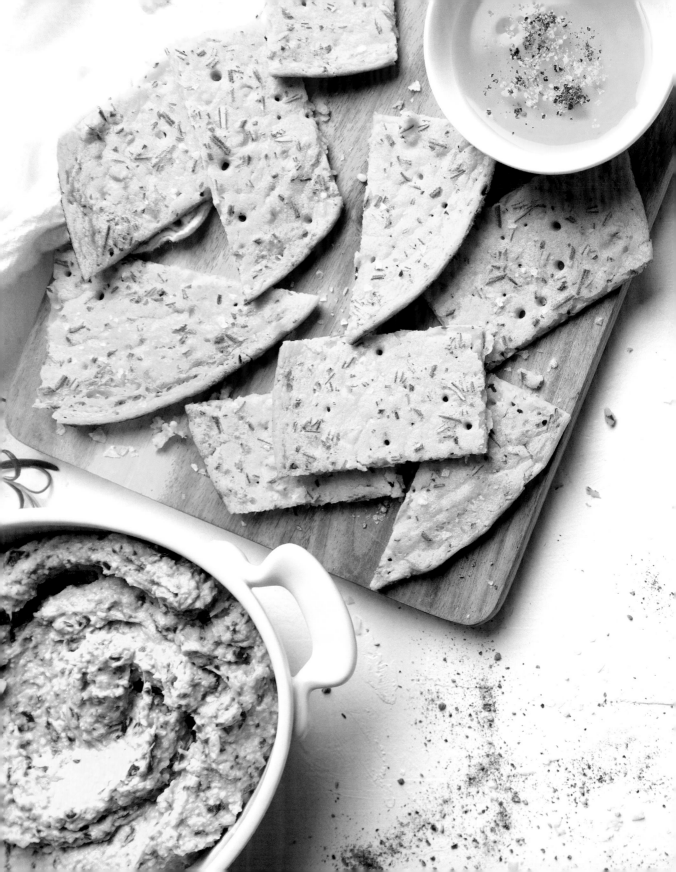

chickpea rosemary flatbread

You may want to go ahead and make two batches of this flatbread—it's that good! Dipped in olive oil or served alongside our Spinach Artichoke Dip, this oh-so-simple bread alternative really hits the spot, and it won't cause gas and bloating like a traditional gluten-filled bread.

Yield **1 thick 10-in flatbread**	Prep Time **10 minutes, plus 1 hour to rest dough**	Cook Time **5 minutes**	80:20

1 cup water

1 cup chickpea flour

2 tbsp minced fresh rosemary

1½ tbsp + 1 tsp olive oil, divided, plus more to serve

½ tsp sea salt, plus more to serve

Freshly ground black pepper, to serve

Spinach Artichoke Dip (optional, page 188), to serve

1. In a small bowl, whisk together the water, chickpea flour, rosemary, 1½ tablespoons oil, and salt. Let the mixture rest for 1 hour to give the flour time to absorb the water.

2. Place an oven rack 6 inches below the broiler. Place a 10- or 12-inch cast-iron skillet on the rack. Turn on the broiler, and allow the skillet to heat for 10 minutes.

3. Carefully remove the hot skillet from the oven. Add the remaining 1 teaspoon oil to coat the bottom of the pan. Whisk the chickpea batter, and pour it into the skillet. Make sure the batter coats the entire surface of the pan.

4. Place under the broiler for 3 to 5 minutes or until the top begins to bubble and brown. The bread should be fairly flexible in the middle but crispy on the edges. Use a spatula to work your way under the bread to remove it from the pan. Slice it into squares, sprinkle with salt and pepper, and drizzle with a good olive oil. Serve on its own or with spinach artichoke dip, if using.

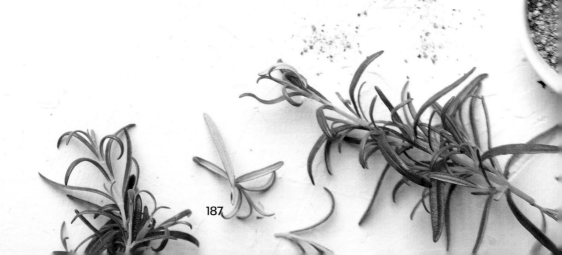

spinach artichoke dip

This recipe was first unveiled on our blog, and the Conscious Cleanse community raved about it. Traditional spinach artichoke dip is loaded with mucus-forming dairy. Our dairy-free version is an irresistibly delicious warm appetizer that's guaranteed to be the hit of the party.

Yield **4 cups**	Prep Time **10 minutes, plus 4-hour soak**	Cook Time **15 minutes**	**CLEANSE**

¾ cup raw cashews, soaked for 4 hours and drained

½ cup water

1 tbsp olive oil

1 small onion, diced

2 cloves garlic, minced

2 (14oz) cans artichoke hearts, drained and rinsed

1 tsp Himalayan pink salt

½ tsp freshly ground black pepper

¼–½ tsp cayenne pepper

2 large handfuls of spinach

½ tbsp freshly squeezed lemon juice

1 cucumber, sliced, to serve

1 In a food processor, blend soaked cashews and water until creamy. Transfer to a small bowl, and set aside. (No need to wash the food processor; you'll use it again in step 3.)

2 In a medium saucepan, heat the oil and onions over low heat, stirring frequently, for 10 minutes or until onions are translucent. Add the garlic and cook for 2 minutes. Stir in the artichokes, salt, black pepper, and cayenne pepper, and heat until warm.

3 Transfer the artichoke mixture to the food processor, and add the spinach, lemon juice, and creamy cashews. Blend until smooth. Serve warm with slices of cucumber.

garlic yam spread

This garlicky vegan spread is one of our favorite fall and wintertime appetizers. It's so good that we could eat it with a spoon—and, in fact, Jules' baby does! Yams are highly nutritious, packed with fiber and antioxidants, and excellent blood sugar stabilizers.

Yield **1½ cups**	Prep Time **5 minutes**	Cook Time **1 hour**	CLEANSE

2 medium yams, pricked with a fork several times

1 head garlic, papery outer layers removed

3 tbsp olive oil, divided

½ tsp Himalayan pink salt

1 Preheat the oven to 400°F, and line a baking sheet with parchment paper. Place the yams on the prepared baking sheet.

2 Cut ¼ to ½ inch from the top of the head of garlic (pointy side), exposing the individual cloves. Place the garlic cut side up on a piece of foil, and drizzle with 1 tablespoon oil, using your fingers to rub the oil into the exposed cloves. Wrap the foil around the garlic, sealing completely. Place on the prepared baking sheet along with the yams.

3 Place the yams and garlic in the oven. After 35 minutes, remove the garlic and let it cool while the yams continue cooking. When cool to the touch, squeeze out 6 cloves. (See tip.) Cook the yams for another 25 minutes (1 hour total) or until tender.

4 When the yams are fully cooked and tender, remove from the oven, and let cool. When cool enough to handle, remove the skins, and place the flesh in a food processor. Add the remaining 2 tablespoons oil, salt, and 6 cloves roasted garlic. Process until smooth and creamy.

5 Serve with Super Seaweed Crackers (page 193) or Golden Flaxseed Crackers (page 192). Store in an airtight container in the refrigerator for up to 5 days.

tip

The remaining roasted garlic can be used as a spread on Golden Flaxseed Crackers or put in a salad dressing.

superfood bars

We're big snackers, so you'll always find us with something stashed in our bags. We created these bars in response to many people's daily reliance on store-bought granola or protein bars. We wanted a bar that was less sweet, packed with more nutrients, and ... wait for it ... a little savory. These are the perfect take-along treat and great for the kids' lunches, so stock up for a quick and easy snack you can feel good about!

Yield **8 bars**	Prep Time **45 minutes**	Cook Time **None**	80:20

¾ cup raw almonds, divided

½ cup raw cashews

4 large Medjool dates, pitted

½ tsp ground cinnamon

1 tbsp cacao powder

2 tbsp melted cacao butter

1–2 tbsp olive oil

2 tbsp chia seeds

2 tbsp hemp seeds

2 tbsp goji berries

¼ cup lightly crumbled store-bought kale chips (plain or sea salt flavor) or homemade kale chips

1 Line an 8 x 8-inch cake pan or baking dish with parchment paper. In a food processor, combine ½ cup raw almonds, cashews, dates, cinnamon, cacao powder, and cacao butter. Pulse until combined. Add the oil 1 tablespoon at a time until the mixture comes together when you squeeze it in your hand.

2 Transfer the mixture to a medium bowl, and add the remaining ¼ cup almonds, chia seeds, hemp seeds, goji berries, and kale chips, stirring to combine.

3 Press the mixture into the prepared pan, and chill in the refrigerator for 30 minutes or until firm. Cut into 6 bars, and store in the refrigerator for up to 1 week.

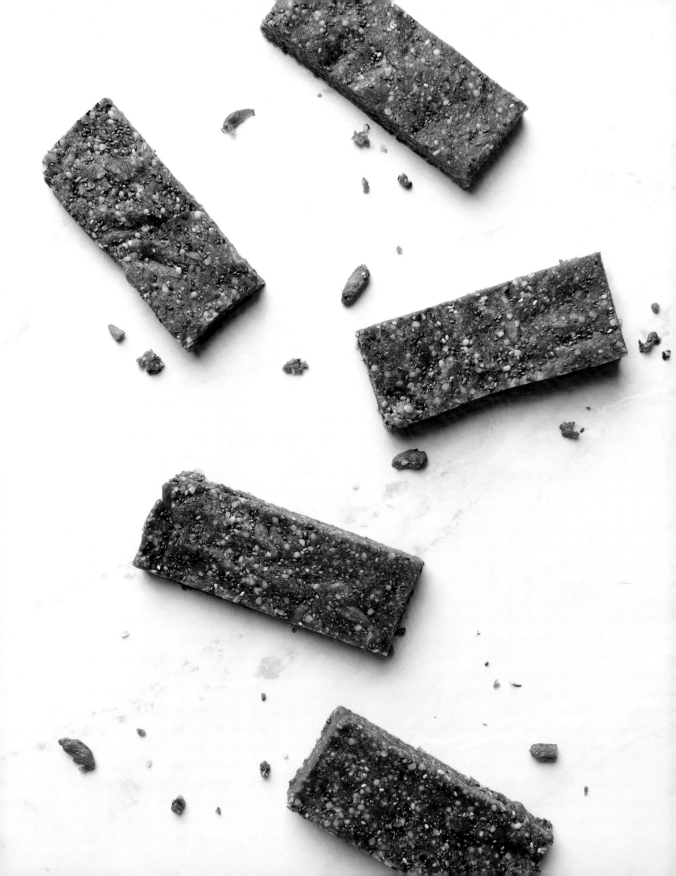

golden flaxseed crackers

Flaxseeds are one of our favorite (and vegan!) ways to get our essential omega-3 fatty acids. They're also packed with plant compounds called lignans, which help to reduce the risk of cancer and balance women's hormones. They're also anti-inflammatory, immune boosting, and critical for a healthy nervous system. Need more to love? Savory and satisfying, these cleanse-friendly crackers deliver the perfect crunch.

Yield **18–20 crackers**	Prep Time **15 minutes**	Cook Time **45 minutes**	CLEANSE

1 cup golden flaxseeds

¼ cup chia seeds

¼ cup sunflower seeds

1 cup warm water

1 cup finely shredded carrots or carrot juice pulp

½ tsp Himalayan pink salt

1 Preheat the oven to 350°F. Line a baking sheet with parchment paper or a silicone liner.

2 In a large bowl, mix together the flaxseeds, chia seeds, sunflower seeds, water, carrots, and salt. Let the mixture sit at room temperature for 10 minutes.

3 Using a spatula, spread the mixture evenly on the prepared baking sheet to a thickness of about ¼ inch. (It will not cover the entire baking sheet.) Bake for 45 minutes or until desired crispness. Let crackers sit for 10 minutes before breaking them apart by hand.

super seaweed crackers

More than a cracker, these Super Seaweed Crackers are packed with plant-based protein, omega-3s, and fiber. The real star of the recipe is seaweed. Naturally salty and high in mighty minerals, these are the cleanse-friendly crackers that our community has been requesting for years.

Yield **18–20 crackers**	Prep Time **10 minutes**	Cook Time **50 minutes**	CLEANSE

1 tbsp arrowroot powder

1 cup boiling water

½ cup brown flaxseeds

3 tbsp black sesame seeds

3 tbsp white sesame seeds

3 tbsp pumpkin seeds

2 tbsp flaked dulse or kelp (Maine Coast Sea Vegetables brand recommended)

1 tsp garlic powder

⅛–¼ tsp cayenne pepper

½ tsp flaky smoked sea salt (Maldon brand recommended)

1 Preheat the oven to 325°F. Line a baking sheet with parchment paper.

2 In a large bowl, whisk together the arrowroot powder and water until there are no clumps. Add the flaxseeds, black and white sesame seeds, pumpkin seeds, dulse, garlic powder, and cayenne. Let the mixture sit for 10 minutes.

3 Using a spatula, spread the mixture evenly on the prepared baking sheet to a thickness of about ¼ inch. (It will not cover the entire baking sheet.) Sprinkle with smoked sea salt, and bake for 45 to 50 minutes or until crispy. Let the crackers sit for 10 to 20 minutes before breaking them apart by hand.

tip

The key to success here is spreading the cracker mixture in a thin, even layer so it bakes evenly and comes out crunchy.

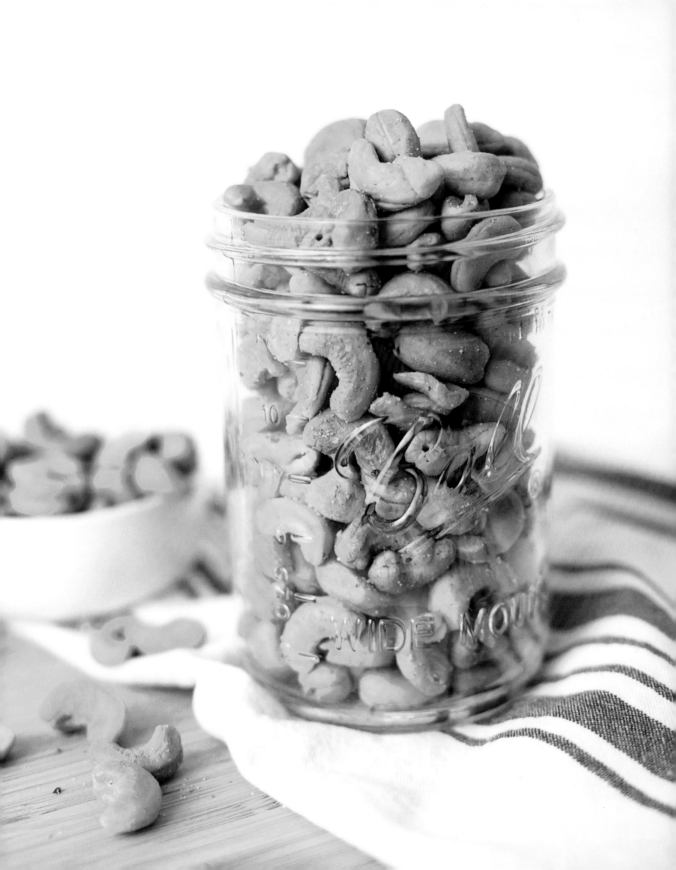

curry roasted cashews

This recipe was contributed by our right-hand woman, Mel, who is the queen of details, all things Instant Pot, and healthy snacking. When she brought these savory cashews to the office one day, we were all hooked.

Yield **2 cups**	Prep Time **5 minutes**	Cook Time **25 minutes**	CLEANSE

1 ½ tbsp coconut oil, melted

2 cups whole raw cashews

1 tsp curry powder

½–1 tsp cayenne pepper

½ tsp Himalayan pink salt

1 Preheat the oven to 275°F. Line a baking sheet with parchment paper or a silicone liner.

2 In a large bowl, combine the melted coconut oil and cashews, stirring until fully coated.

3 In a small bowl, mix together the curry powder, cayenne, and salt. Add the spice mixture to the cashews, and stir until fully coated.

4 Spread the cashews on the prepared baking sheet, and roast for 25 minutes. Remove from the oven and let cool. Refrigerate in an airtight container for up to 2 weeks. (As the coconut oil cools, a white film may appear on the nuts.)

roasted chickpeas

Ah, the mighty chickpea! So delicious, high in protein, and extremely versatile. We love adding savory roasted chickpeas to soups and salads for extra crunch, while our kiddos love the sweet variation packed in their lunches. Perfect by the handful for a healthy and filling plant-powered snack.

Yield **3 cups**	Prep Time **5 minutes**	Cook Time **35–40 minutes**	CLEANSE

2 (15oz) cans chickpeas, drained and rinsed

2 tbsp olive oil

Seasoning mixture of choice

Garlic and Onion

1 tsp garlic powder

½ tsp onion powder

½ tsp Himalayan pink salt

Cinnamon and "Sugar"

1 tsp cinnamon

1 tbsp Lakanto Classic Monkfruit Sweetener

½ tsp Himalayan pink salt

Curry and Cayenne

1 tsp curry powder

½–1 tsp cayenne pepper

½ tsp Himalayan pink salt

1 Preheat the oven to 400°F. Line a baking sheet with parchment paper. Pat the chickpeas with a paper towel to dry.

2 In a large bowl, combine the chickpeas, oil, and seasoning mixture of your choice. Toss to coat evenly. Spread the chickpeas in an even layer on the prepared baking sheet, and bake for 35 to 40 minutes or until crispy. Remove from the oven, and adjust salt to taste.

3 To store, cool completely and place in an airtight container in the refrigerator for up to 7 days.

tip

Did you know that the liquid from a can of chickpeas (called aquafaba) makes a perfect egg replacement? To make 1 aquafaba "egg," reserve 3 tablespoons liquid from canned chickpeas. Whisk vigorously until foamy, and use in place of 1 egg. Just another reason to love the mighty chickpea!

parsnip fries

One of Jo's personal favorites, parsnip fries are so fun to eat, they're a must when you're on the Conscious Cleanse. Once you master this recipe, feel free to switch it up with the almighty sweet potato or humble carrot. To ensure a crispy fry, be sure to let them breathe, keeping plenty of space between each fry.

Yield **4 servings**	Prep Time **20 minutes**	Cook Time **30–40 minutes**	CLEANSE

2½ lb parsnips (about 6 large parsnips)

2 tbsp olive oil

Himalayan pink salt and freshly ground black pepper, to taste

2 tbsp chopped fresh Italian (flat-leaf) parsley, to garnish

½ tsp paprika (optional)

1 Preheat the oven to 425°F. Line two baking sheets with parchment paper. Trim and peel the parsnips, and cut them into ½-inch thick "fries."

2 In a large bowl, toss the parsnips with oil to coat. Arrange the parsnips on the prepared baking sheets in a single layer, evenly spaced. Bake for 30 to 40 minutes (depending on how crispy you like your fries), flipping the parsnips and rotating the trays halfway through cooking.

3 Remove from the oven and sprinkle with salt and pepper. Garnish with parsley and paprika, if using.

sesame cauli wings

If you love sesame chicken from your favorite Chinese restaurant, you'll love our meatless makeover featuring cauliflower. The secret sauce is just as sweet, sticky, and lip-smacking good as the original.

Yield **2–4 servings**	Prep Time **20 minutes**	Cook Time **35 minutes**	80:20

1 cup cassava flour

½ tsp garlic powder

¼ tsp Himalayan pink salt

1¼ cups water

1 head cauliflower, cut into florets (about 4 cups)

2½ tsp toasted sesame oil, divided

1-in piece fresh ginger, peeled and minced

2–3 cloves garlic, minced

3 tbsp honey

2½ tbsp coconut aminos

1 tsp rice vinegar

1 tsp chili paste

2 tbsp sesame seeds, to garnish

¼ cup sliced scallions, to garnish

1 Preheat the oven to 425°F. Line two baking sheets with parchment paper.

2 In a large bowl, combine the cassava flour, garlic powder, and salt. Add the water, and stir until a pancake-like batter consistency is reached. Toss the cauliflower florets in the batter, and stir to combine.

3 One at a time, shake off the excess batter and place the battered florets on the prepared baking sheets, leaving enough room between the florets for them to get crispy. Bake for 20 minutes, rotate the trays (switching trays from top to bottom racks), and bake for 10 to 15 more minutes or until crispy and browned.

4 Meanwhile, in a small saucepan, heat 2 teaspoons sesame oil over medium-low heat. Add the ginger and garlic, and sauté for 60 seconds or until fragrant, stirring frequently. Add the honey, coconut aminos, rice vinegar, and chili paste, and stir well. Continue cooking over medium-low heat, stirring frequently, for about 5 minutes. The sauce should thicken slightly. Stir in the remaining ½ teaspoon sesame oil just before mixing with the cauliflower.

5 When the cauliflower is done baking, transfer it to a large bowl, pour the sauce over it, and gently mix until fully coated. Transfer the cauliflower back to the baking sheets, and bake for 2 to 4 minutes to set the sauce onto the cauliflower. Remove from the oven and garnish with sesame seeds and scallions. Serve immediately.

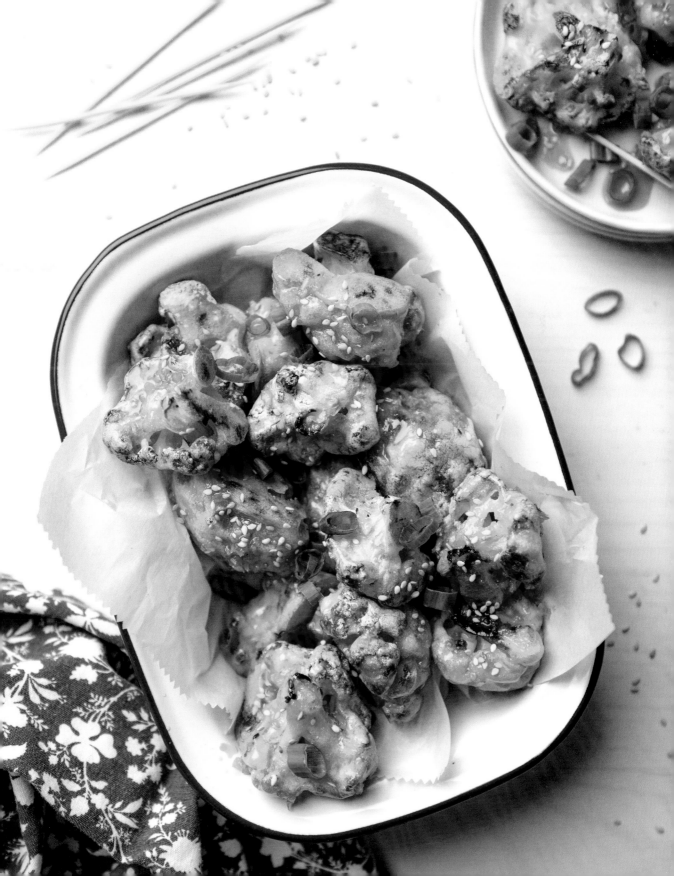

sweet treats

peach crumble bars 202

carob chia pudding 204

five-spice pumpkin cookies 205

cashew cupcakes.. 207

vanilla tiger nut cupcakes 208

molten chocolate cake.. 210

chocolate dessert hummus 212

greensicle popsicles 213

chocolate tahini energy balls 215

zesty lemon balls 216

chocolate chip cookie dough balls 217

no-bake mini carrot cake bites 218

vanilla almond macaroons 220

sunflower cookies.. 221

pumpkin fudge 223

carob hazelnut cheesecake 224

salted caramel ice cream 225

chocolate chickpea ice cream 226

peach crumble bars

We created these bars at the height of peach season in Colorado, resulting in the perfect BBQ treat or kid-friendly snack. Part of their charm is they're super simple to make and you can swap out the peaches for any fresh fruit that's in season.

Yield **12 bars**	Prep Time **15 minutes**	Cook Time **30 minutes**	80:20

For the crust and topping

1½ cups almond flour

¼ cup brown rice flour

2 tbsp ground flaxseeds

1 tsp baking powder

1 tsp ground cinnamon

½ tsp Himalayan pink salt

½ cup almond butter

6 tbsp maple syrup

½ tsp pure almond extract

For the filling

3–4 peaches, peeled and chopped (about 3 cups; see note)

3 tbsp maple syrup

1 tbsp chia seeds

½ tsp pure almond extract

1 Preheat the oven to 350°F, and line an 8 x 8-inch baking dish with two pieces of parchment paper, one going in each direction.

2 To make the crust and topping, in a large bowl, whisk together the almond flour, brown rice flour, ground flaxseeds, baking powder, cinnamon, and salt. In a small bowl, mix together the almond butter, maple syrup, and almond extract. Add the wet mixture to the dry mixture, and stir until thoroughly combined. (It should be wet enough to hold together well and not crumble apart.) Reserve ½ cup packed dough and set aside. Press the remaining dough into the prepared pan. Smooth it out, and bake for 8 minutes. Remove from the oven and set aside to cool.

3 To make the filling, in a medium saucepan, heat the peaches and maple syrup over medium-high heat. Bring to a low boil. When boiling, reduce heat to medium-low. Simmer for 10 minutes, stirring frequently. Stir in the chia seeds, and cook for 5 minutes or until thickened. Remove from heat and stir in the almond extract.

4 To assemble, spread the peach filling over the almond crust, and carefully smooth it out. Crumble the reserved dough over top. Bake at 350°F for 12 to 13 minutes, watching closely to ensure it does not burn. The crumble topping will be golden when ready. Cool in the pan on a wire rack before cutting, about 30 to 45 minutes.

note

If fresh peaches aren't available, you can substitute frozen peaches. Just be sure to thaw and drain well before chopping.

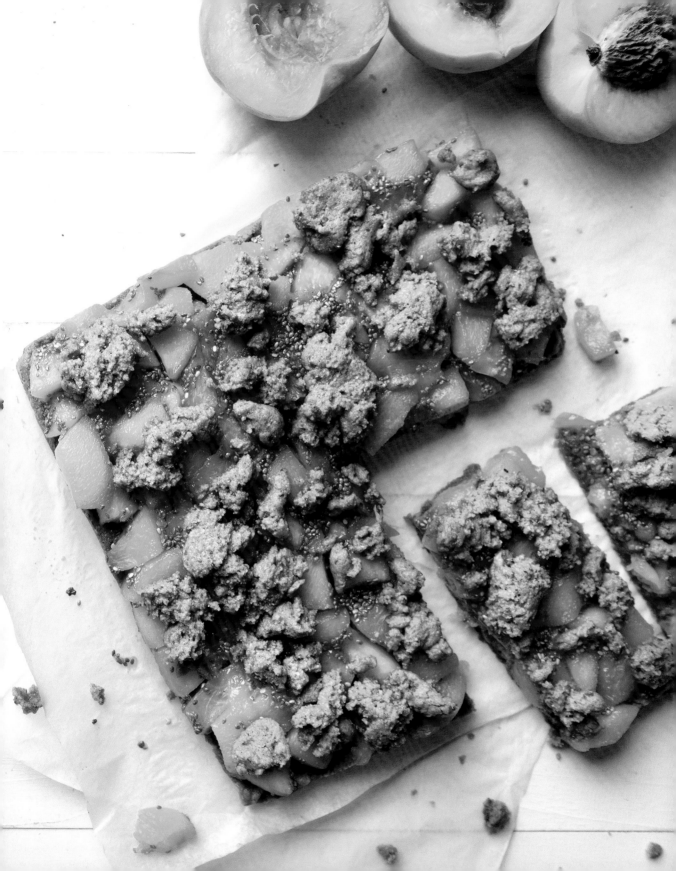

carob chia pudding

Better than chocolate pudding, this treat checks all the boxes: rich in protein, dairy-free, and perfect for our Low Sugar Track. We love chia seeds, which are loaded with antioxidants, omega-3 fatty acids, and fiber.

Yield **4 servings**	Prep Time **5 minutes, plus 6 hours to set**	Cook Time **None**	**LS** CLEANSE

1 (13.5oz) can full-fat coconut milk

½ cup **Almond Milk** (page 230)

¼ cup chia seeds

½ cup carob powder

½ tsp pure vanilla extract

Pinch of Himalayan pink salt

1 tsp Lakanto Classic Monkfruit Sweetener, or 4 tsp stevia (optional)

Unsweetened coconut flakes (optional), to garnish

Fresh berries (optional), to garnish

1. In a high-speed blender, combine the coconut milk, almond milk, chia seeds, carob powder, vanilla, salt, and sweetener, if using. Blend until smooth.

2. Pour the mixture into four small Mason jars, cover, and refrigerate overnight or for at least 6 hours. Serve garnished with coconut flakes or berries, if using.

variation
Feel free to substitute raw cacao powder for the carob when not cleansing.

five-spice pumpkin cookies

These delicious, low-sugar cookies feature five-spice powder, which represents the five flavors—sour, bitter, sweet, pungent, and salty. When paired with pumpkin and tiger nut flour, the result is a fiber-rich, nutrient-dense cookie that will delight all of your senses. Enjoy with our Turmeric Tonic Latte.

Yield **24 cookies**	Prep Time **10 minutes**	Cook Time **12 minutes**	80:20

1 cup tiger nut flour

¼ cup cassava flour

1 tsp baking soda

1 tbsp five-spice powder

5 tbsp Lakanto Classic Monkfruit Sweetener

½ tsp Himalayan pink salt

1 egg (see note)

¼ cup palm shortening

1 tsp pure vanilla extract

½ cup pumpkin purée

3 tbsp dairy-free chocolate chips (Enjoy Life brand recommended)

1. Preheat the oven to 350°F. Line a baking sheet with parchment paper or a silicone liner.

2. In a small bowl, mix together the tiger nut flour, cassava flour, baking soda, five-spice powder, sweetener, and salt.

3. In a medium bowl, whisk together the egg, palm shortening, vanilla, and pumpkin purée.

4. Add the dry ingredients to the wet ingredients, and mix until fully incorporated. Stir in the chocolate chips.

5. Using a cookie scoop, place 1-inch cookie dough balls on the prepared baking sheet. Bake for 10 to 12 minutes. Remove from the oven and let cool on the baking sheet.

variation

Make egg-free using one of these egg stubstitutes.

For flax egg: In a small bowl, whisk 1 tablespoon ground flaxseeds with 3 tablespoons water. Let sit for 10 minutes at room temperature. Use in place of 1 egg.

For aquafaba egg: Reserve 3 tablespoons of liquid from canned chickpeas. Whisk vigorously until foamy, and use in place of 1 egg.

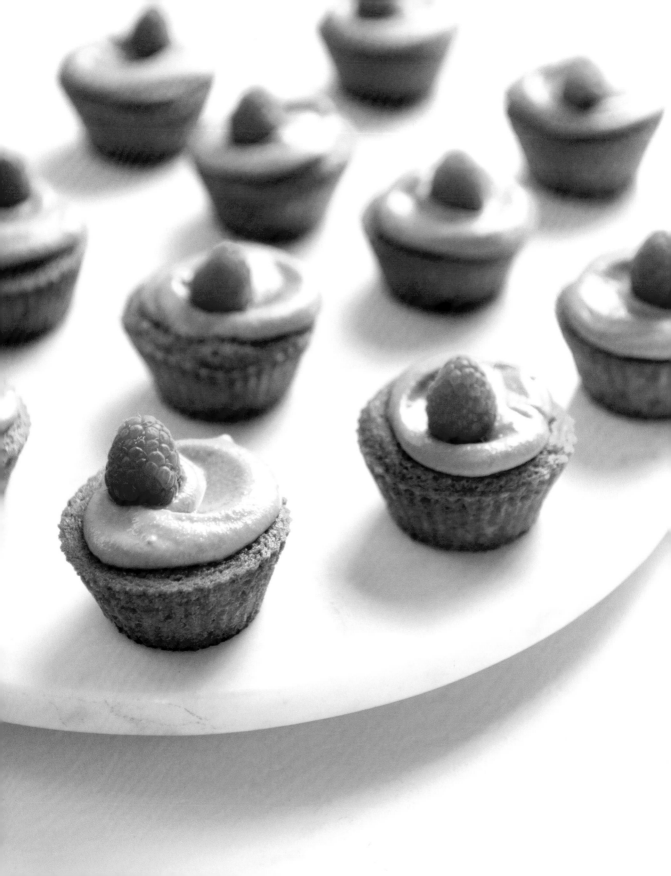

cashew cupcakes
WITH FRESH RASPBERRY FROSTING

Perfect for your next celebration, these cupcakes are light, fluffy, and not too sweet. Many grain-free baked goods feature almonds, but we've found that some people have developed a sensitivity to almonds from eating them too often. That's why we love rotating in cashew flour as a healthy alternative to almond flour whenever possible.

Yield **9 cupcakes**	Prep Time **15 minutes, plus 1-hour soak**	Cook Time **30 minutes**	80:20

2 cups cashew flour

¼ tsp Himalayan pink salt

½ tsp baking soda

2 eggs

½ cup full-fat coconut milk

½ cup maple syrup (or Lakanto Classic Monkfruit Sweetener for low sugar)

For the frosting

1¼ cups raw cashews, soaked for 1 hour, drained and rinsed

1 cup fresh raspberries, plus more to garnish

¼ cup coconut cream (from 1 can full-fat coconut milk that has been refrigerated overnight)

¼ cup maple syrup

1 tbsp coconut oil, melted

1 tsp pure vanilla extract

½ tbsp freshly squeezed lemon juice

¼ tsp Himalayan pink salt

1 Preheat the oven to 350°F. Line a 12-cup muffin pan with 9 liners (paper or silicone).

2 In a large bowl, stir together the cashew flour, salt, and baking soda. In a small bowl, whisk together the eggs, coconut milk, and maple syrup until well combined.

3 Slowly add the wet ingredients to the dry ingredients, and stir to combine. Scoop batter into each liner, filling them about ¾ full. Bake for 25 to 30 minutes or until a toothpick inserted into the center of a cupcake comes out clean. Allow to cool for at least 1 hour before frosting.

4 To make the frosting, in a high-speed blender, combine the cashews, raspberries, coconut cream (the top layer of chilled coconut milk; reserve the leftover liquid for a smoothie), maple syrup, oil, vanilla, lemon juice, and salt. Blend until creamy. Refrigerate until ready to use.

5 When the cupcakes are fully cooled, top with frosting and garnish with fresh berries. Cupcakes can be refrigerated in an airtight glass container for up to 5 days.

vanilla tiger nut cupcakes

Finding a sweet treat that's healthy, low in sugar, grain-free, and nut-free is a tall order. This cupcake delivers, with two different decadent frosting options to boot! Egg-free and naturally sweetened with ripe bananas, this is a dessert for everyone. We love baking with protein- and fiber-rich tiger nut flour, which doesn't come from a nut as the name suggests, but from a small root vegetable.

Yield **24 cupcakes or 48 mini cupcakes**	Prep Time **10 minutes**	Cook Time **30 minutes**	80:20

6 ripe bananas, mashed with a fork

10 tbsp Lakanto Classic Monkfruit Sweetener

1 tbsp pure vanilla extract

½ cup aquafaba (liquid from canned chickpeas), whipped (see note)

4 cups tiger nut flour

2 tbsp baking powder

1 tbsp ground cinnamon

½ tsp Himalayan pink salt

1. Preheat the oven to 350°F. Line two 12-cup muffin pans or two 24-cup mini muffin pans with paper liners.

2. In a medium bowl, combine the mashed bananas, sweetener, and vanilla. Stir until smooth. Add the whipped aquafaba, and mix again until smooth.

3. In a large bowl, whisk together the tiger nut flour, baking powder, cinnamon, and salt. Pour the wet mixture over the dry mixture, and stir until combined and no dry streaks remain.

4. Scoop the batter into the prepared muffin cups, filling them ¾ full. Bake for 25 to 30 (regular cupcakes) or 15 minutes (mini cupcakes), or until a skewer comes out clean. Let cool completely before topping with Carob Avocado Frosting or Coconut Cream Frosting.

note

To prepare the aquafaba, pour the liquid from 1 (15oz) can chickpeas into a medium bowl. (Reserve the beans for another use.) With a whisk, whip the liquid for 3 to 4 minutes or until slightly foamy.

CAROB AVOCADO FROSTING

Yield **3 cups**
Prep Time **10 minutes**
Cook Time **None**

1½ large ripe avocados

5 tbsp roasted carob powder

1½ ripe bananas

¼ tsp Himalayan pink salt

1 tbsp pure vanilla extract

1 In a high-speed blender, combine the avocados, carob powder, bananas, salt, and vanilla. Blend until smooth and creamy.

2 If needed, add a little water to thin the mixture to a spreadable consistency, but take care not to add too much. It spreads best when still creamy. Spread on cupcakes, swirling the tops.

COCONUT CREAM FROSTING

Yield **3 cups**
Prep Time **10 minutes**
Cook Time **None**

3 (5.4oz) cans coconut cream, refrigerated overnight

1 tbsp pure vanilla extract

Unsweetened shredded coconut, to garnish

1 Open the cans of coconut cream, and separate the solid portion from the liquid. Reserve the liquid for another use (like your morning green smoothie).

2 Using a mixer, beat the solid coconut cream and vanilla on medium speed until thick and creamy. Spread on cupcakes, and top with unsweetened shredded coconut.

molten chocolate cake
WITH COCONUT WHIPPED CREAM

Flourless chocolate cake oozing with dark chocolate? Sign us up! These sexy little chocolate cakes are perfect for your next romantic encounter or when you want to impress your dinner party guests.

Yield **4 servings**	Prep Time **15 minutes**	Cook Time **20 minutes**	80:20

¼ cup coconut oil, plus more to grease ramekins (or olive oil)

2 tbsp raw cacao powder, plus more for dusting

1½ tbsp almond flour

¼ tsp Himalayan pink salt

6 oz 88% dark chocolate

3 eggs

3 tbsp maple syrup

1 tsp pure vanilla extract

Fresh raspberries (optional), to serve

For the whipped cream (optional)

1 (13.5oz) can full-fat coconut milk, refrigerated overnight

1½ tbsp honey

1½ tsp pure vanilla extract

1 Preheat the oven to 375°F. Lightly grease four ramekins with oil, then dust each one with a pinch of cacao powder.

2 In a small bowl, mix together the remaining cacao powder, almond flour, and salt. Set aside.

3 In a small saucepan, melt the remaining ¼ cup coconut oil and dark chocolate over low heat, stirring continuously, being careful not to burn or get too hot.

4 In a medium bowl, whisk together the eggs, maple syrup, and vanilla until frothy. Pour the melted chocolate mixture into the bowl, and stir to combine.

5 Add the almond flour mixture to the bowl with the wet ingredients, and stir to combine. Divide the batter evenly among the four ramekins, and place the ramekins on a baking sheet. Bake on the center rack for 10 to 12 minutes.

6 Meanwhile, to make the whipped cream, if using, carefully open the can of refrigerated coconut milk. Keeping the can level, scrape out the thick top layer of coconut cream, and place it in a medium bowl. Using a mixer on high speed, whip the coconut cream for 3 minutes or until it becomes light and fluffy. Add the honey and vanilla, and beat for 2 minutes more.

7 Serve in the ramekins, or allow cakes to cool before removing them from the ramekins. Top with coconut whipped cream and berries, if using, and another dusting of cacao powder.

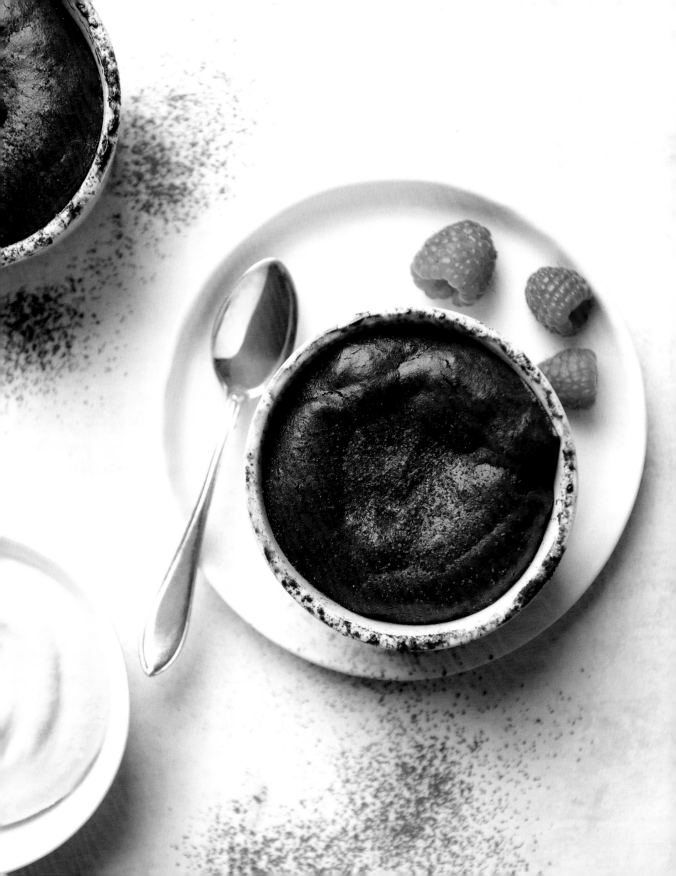

chocolate dessert hummus

Want your kids to snack on more veggies? This sweet, dessert-like hummus gets the job done! Chocolate hummus may sound unexpected, but trust us when we say that this combination works. Chickpeas, raw cacao, and a little maple syrup make for a guilt-free, protein-rich, decadent dip.

Yield **2 cups**	Prep Time **15 minutes**	Cook Time **None**	80:20

1 (15oz) can chickpeas, drained and rinsed

¼ raw tahini (Artisana Organics brand recommended)

½ cup raw cacao powder

½ cup maple syrup

1 tsp pure vanilla extract

½ tsp Himalayan pink salt

2 tbsp water, to thin

1 In a food processor, combine the chickpeas, tahini, cacao powder, maple syrup, vanilla, and salt. Blend until smooth and creamy, adding a little water at a time only if necessary to reach desired consistency.

2 Refrigerate in an airtight container for up to 1 week. Serve with carrots, celery, fruit, or rice crackers.

greensicle popsicles

Homemade popsicles are a must-try if you have kids—no need to tell them that you put spinach and avocado in them! This is one of our favorite variations because it's hydrating and packed with vitamin C, but you can really put any green smoothie recipe into an ice pop mold for a fun summertime treat.

Yield **6 popsicles**	Prep Time **15 minutes, plus 8 hours to freeze**	Cook Time **None**	80:20

1 cup plain coconut water

2 oranges, peeled

1 banana, frozen

1 vanilla bean, scraped

½ avocado, frozen (see tip)

1 cup spinach, packed

1 In a high-speed blender, combine the coconut water, oranges, banana, and vanilla. Blend until smooth.

2 Pour ¾ of the mixture evenly into six BPA-free ice pop molds to make the first layer of the popsicles (the orange layer).

3 Add the avocado and spinach to the remaining mixture in the blender, and blend until smooth. Pour evenly into the ice pop molds. (This will create a green layer.) Freeze overnight.

4 To release the ice pops from the molds, run under hot water until you can wiggle them free.

tip
Never waste a ripe avocado again! Just scoop the flesh out and store in an airtight container in the freezer. Perfect for green smoothies or popsicles.

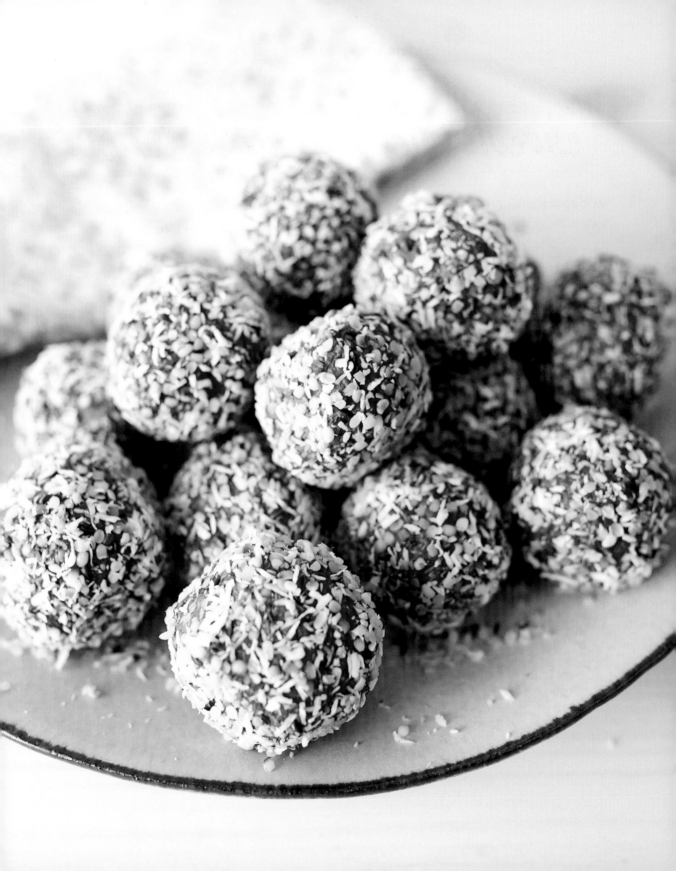

chocolate tahini energy balls

We're big fans of raw balls because they're a healthy snack that packs a mighty, nutrient-dense punch. Nutty tahini and rich chocolate will satisfy your sweet tooth and keep you feeling full all afternoon long. Store in the freezer for a portable burst of energy that you can take anywhere.

| Yield **16 balls** | Prep Time **15 minutes, plus 20 minutes to chill** | Cook Time **None** | 80:20 |

1 cup + 2 tbsp unsweetened shredded coconut, divided

4 tbsp melted cacao butter

½ cup raw tahini (Artisana Organics brand recommended)

½ cup Medjool dates, pitted (about 5 dates)

¼ cup cacao powder

Pinch of Himalayan pink salt

¼ cup unsweetened cacao nibs

2 tbsp hemp seeds

1 In a food processor, combine 1 cup shredded coconut, cacao butter, tahini, dates, cacao powder, and salt. Process for about 1 minute or until a smooth texture forms.

2 Transfer the mixture to a medium bowl, and stir in the cacao nibs. Place the mixture in the refrigerator to chill for 20 minutes.

3 In a small bowl, combine the hemp seeds and remaining 2 tablespoons shredded coconut.

4 Using your hands, form the coconut-tahini mixture into about 16 (1-inch) balls. Roll the balls in the coconut hemp seed mixture to coat, and place in a container with a tight-fitting lid. Store in the freezer or refrigerator. Enjoy chilled or frozen.

tip

For several different cleanse-friendly raw ball recipes, be sure to check out our blog at consciouscleanse.com.

zesty lemon balls

We love a good recipe challenge, so when a friend asked us for a lemon bar that wasn't packed with sugar, butter, eggs, and gluten, we gladly accepted. These tasty bites are the result, and they sing of summertime. Featuring macadamia nuts, these are a protein-packed dessert, perfect for your next picnic.

Yield **16 balls**	Prep Time **15 minutes**	Cook Time **None**	80:20

¼ cup macadamia nuts

1½ cups almond flour

1 tbsp coconut flour

¼ cup + 2 tbsp freshly squeezed lemon juice

3 tbsp honey

¼ cup coconut oil, melted

2 tsp pure vanilla extract

1 tsp lemon zest

¼ tsp Himalayan pink salt

½ cup shredded coconut

1 In a food processor, pulse the macadamia nuts until fine. Add the almond flour, coconut flour, lemon juice, honey, oil, vanilla, lemon zest, and salt. Pulse again until well combined.

2 Spread the shredded coconut on a plate. Using your hands, form the nut and honey mixture into 16 balls (about 2 tablespoons each), and roll each ball in coconut to coat.

3 Store in an airtight container and freeze or refrigerate until ready to serve.

chocolate chip cookie dough balls

Kudos to the person who first thought of making cookie dough a thing of its own! Featuring tiger nut flour, these are one of our favorite sweet treats. They're quick to whip together and dangerously delicious.

Yield **12 balls**	Prep Time **5 minutes**	Cook Time **None**	80:20

1½ cups tiger nut flour

¼ tsp Himalayan pink salt

2 tbsp raw honey or maple syrup

1½ tsp pure vanilla extract

4 tbsp olive oil

4–6 tbsp dairy-free mini chocolate chips (Enjoy Life brand recommended) or cacao nibs

1 In a medium bowl, combine the tiger nut flour, salt, honey, vanilla, and oil. Using your hands or the back of a wooden spoon, rub all the ingredients together until they form a coarse meal and are distributed evenly. Add the chocolate chips or cacao nibs, and mix.

2 Scoop a heaping tablespoon of the mixture, and roll until it holds together into a ball. (You may need to add a splash more oil to get the mixture to the correct consistency.) Store in the refrigerator or freezer for up to 1 week.

variation

If you don't have tiger nut flour on hand, almond flour makes an excellent substitute. Also, melted coconut oil can be used in place of the olive oil with equally delicious results.

no-bake mini carrot cake bites

In college, Jules worked at a bakery, and during that time she was on a strict carrot cake diet. (Something we do not recommend!) This raw treat transforms a sugar- and gluten-filled gut bomb and takes it to another, superfood level. Quick and easy, this is the perfect bite-sized dessert for picnics or gatherings.

Yield **9 bites**	Prep Time **15 minutes, plus overnight soak**	Cook Time **None**	80:20

⅓ cup pecans

⅓ cup walnuts

⅓ cup cashews

1 cup Medjool dates, pitted

½ cup shredded carrot

1 tsp ground cinnamon, plus more for dusting

½ tsp ground nutmeg

¼ tsp Himalayan pink salt

For the frosting

½ cup raw cashews, soaked overnight and drained

2 tbsp freshly squeezed lemon juice

¼ tsp lemon zest

1 tsp maple syrup

½ tbsp Lakanto Classic Monkfruit Sweetener

½ tsp pure vanilla extract

Pinch of Himalayan pink salt, or to taste

2–4 tbsp water, based on desired thickness

1 In a food processor, pulse the pecans, walnuts, and cashews until fine. Add the dates, carrots, cinnamon, nutmeg, and salt, and combine well. Line an 8 x 8-inch cake pan with parchment paper. Press the mixture into the prepared pan, and smooth. Place in the refrigerator to chill while you make the frosting.

2 To make the frosting, in a small high-speed blender, combine the cashews, lemon juice, lemon zest, maple syrup, sweetener, vanilla, salt, and 2 tablespoons water. Blend until creamy. Scrape down the sides and add more water if needed to achieve a creamy, spreadable texture.

3 Remove the carrot cake from the refrigerator, and spread the frosting evenly over top. Return to the refrigerator for at least 1 hour to chill before cutting into bite-sized squares. Dust with cinnamon before serving.

tip
A small blender, such as a NutriBullet, or a mini food processor work best for the frosting.

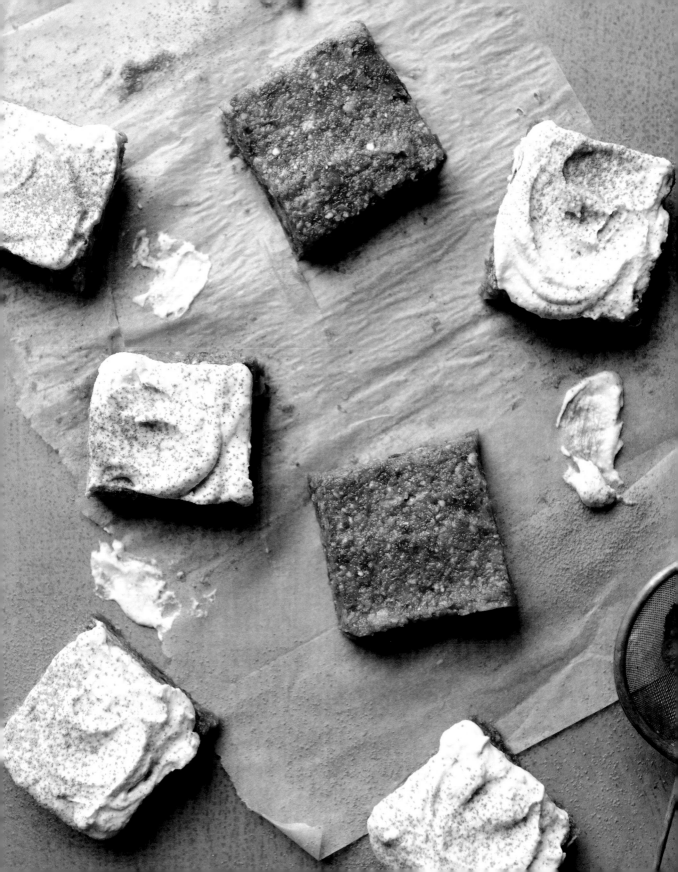

vanilla almond macaroons
WITH CHOCOLATE DRIZZLE

Coconut macaroons are typically loaded with sugar, milk, and eggs. Our nearly raw, vegan version is stripped down to simple, wholesome ingredients with an optional chocolate drizzle that gives "almond joy" a whole new meaning. Looking for more chocolate? Be sure to try the dark chocolate variation!

Yield **24 macaroons**	Prep Time **20 minutes**	Cook Time **25 minutes**	80:20

¾ cup maple syrup

½ cup coconut butter, melted

1 tsp pure vanilla extract

1 tsp pure almond extract

3 cups unsweetened shredded coconut

1½ cups almond flour

½ tsp Himalayan pink salt

For the chocolate drizzle (optional)

½ cup finely grated cacao butter

1 tbsp coconut oil

¼ cup raw cacao powder

3 tbsp maple syrup

1 Preheat the oven to 325°F. Line a baking sheet with parchment paper.

2 In a large bowl, combine the maple syrup, coconut butter, vanilla extract, and almond extract. Stir until creamy. Add the coconut, almond flour, and salt, and stir until fully combined. (It may take some muscle.) You can also use your hands to get the mixture fully incorporated.

3 Using a small ice cream scoop, spoon the dough onto the prepared baking sheet. Place in the oven for 20 to 25 minutes. Remove and let cool.

4 To make the chocolate drizzle, if using, in a small saucepan, melt the cacao butter and oil over low heat. Add the cacao powder and maple syrup, and stir continuously until fully incorporated. Drizzle over top of the macaroons (or dip them right in!).

5 To store, refrigerate or freeze in an airtight container.

variation

For Dark Chocolate Macaroons, omit the almond extract and add 1½ cups raw cacao powder with the coconut in step 2.

sunflower cookies

Our take on traditional peanut butter blossom cookies, these cookies skip all the gluten and sugar. Swapping out peanut butter for sunflower seed butter results in a delicious treat for those with nut allergies. Chock-full of healthy fats and protein, this is a cookie you can feel good about giving your kids!

	Yield **20 cookies**	Prep Time **20 minutes**	Cook Time **15 minutes**	80:20

1 egg

1 cup unsweetened sunflower seed butter

1 tsp pure vanilla extract

½ cup maple syrup

¾ cup cassava flour

½ tsp Himalayan pink salt, plus more for finishing

1 Preheat the oven to 350°F, and line a baking sheet with parchment paper. In a large bowl, whisk the egg and then add the sunflower seed butter, vanilla, and maple syrup. Stir until fully incorporated. Add the cassava flour and salt, and stir to combine.

2 Using a cookie scoop, place 1-inch cookie dough balls on the prepared baking sheet. Use a fork to flatten and imprint a crosshatch on each cookie. Bake for 10 to 15 minutes or until the cookies are golden brown. Remove from the oven, and sprinkle with a pinch of salt.

tip

Instead of sprinkling with Himalayan pink salt in step 2, try Maldon smoked sea salt for a delicious smoky flavor or Lakanto Classic Monkfruit Sweetener for added sweetness.

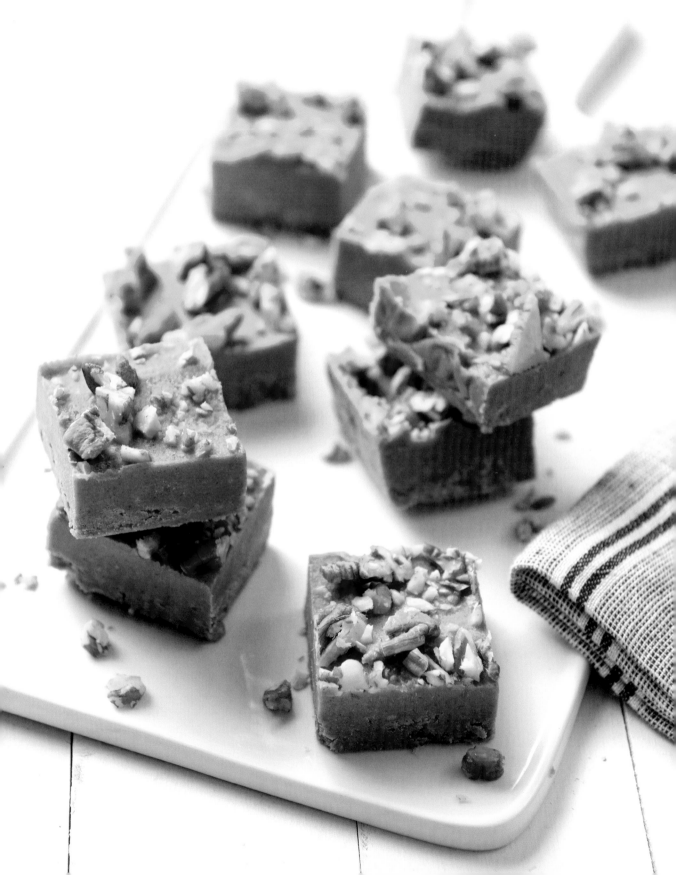

pumpkin fudge

What's better than pumpkin pie? Pumpkin fudge! Our version is vegan, rich, and decadent—and it takes less than 30 minutes to prepare. The star of the recipe is the lucuma powder, which is a low-glycemic superfood sweetener that's packed with fiber.

Yield **24 1-inch pieces**	Prep Time **15 minutes, plus 4 hours to chill**	Cook Time **3 minutes**	80:20

½ cup canned pumpkin purée

⅓ cup almond butter

3 tbsp lucuma powder

3 tbsp maple syrup

½ tsp ground cinnamon

Pinch of Himalayan pink salt

⅓ cup coconut butter

3 tbsp coconut oil

Cacao nibs (optional), for topping

Pecans, finely chopped (optional), for topping

1 In a medium bowl, combine the pumpkin, almond butter, lucuma powder, maple syrup, cinnamon, and salt. Stir until smooth.

2 In a small saucepan, melt together the coconut butter and oil over low heat. Pour the coconut mixture into the pumpkin mixture, and stir to combine.

3 Line a loaf pan with plastic wrap, and press the mixture into the prepared pan. Sprinkle with cacao nibs, if using, for an extra chocolaty crunch or pecans, for a nutty flavor. Place in the freezer for 3 to 4 hours. When ready to serve, cut into small pieces. Store in an airtight container in the freezer.

carob hazelnut cheesecake

This decadent dessert was first featured at one of our community-based "cleanse-time" dinners in our hometown of Boulder, Colorado. Using only cleanse-approved ingredients, this recipe features carob, a sweet and healthy alternative to chocolate that's rich in antioxidants and naturally caffeine-free, unlike its chocolaty friends, cocoa and cacao.

Yield **8–10 servings**	Prep Time **20 minutes , plus 4-hour soak and overnight freeze**	Cook Time **None**	CLEANSE

For the crust

½ cup hazelnuts

½ cup pecans

½ cup Medjool dates, pitted and soaked for at least 15 minutes

¼ cup shredded coconut

Pinch of Himalayan pink salt

For the filling

3 cups raw cashews, soaked for at least 4 hours and drained

⅔ cup maple syrup or honey

½ cup freshly squeezed lemon juice

¾ cup coconut oil, melted

¾ cup carob powder

2 tsp pure vanilla extract

¼ cup water

1 To make the crust, in a food processor, process the hazelnuts and pecans until fine. Add the dates, coconut, and salt, and process until well combined. Transfer to a 9-inch round cake pan and, using your hands, press down to spread the mixture evenly over the bottom of the pan. Place in the freezer until ready to use.

2 To make the filling, in a food processor or high-speed blender, process the cashews, maple syrup or honey, lemon juice, oil, carob powder, and vanilla until well combined. Add the water slowly (you may not need to use all of it) until you reach your desired consistency. It should be nice and creamy. Pour into the crust, and place back in the freezer overnight. Serve cold.

variation

Not a fan of carob? Replace it with raw cacao powder for a more traditional chocolate cheesecake when not cleansing.

salted caramel ice cream

The combination of salt and caramel is truly a match made in heaven. And that's what we have here with this dairy-free, cashew-based "nice" cream. Regular ice cream can cause bloating, gas, and stuffy sinuses. Now you can enjoy this creamy, decadent combo all summer without the unwanted side effects.

| Yield **8 servings** | Prep Time **15 minutes, plus 2-hour soak and overnight freeze** | Cook Time **None** | 80:20 |

3 cups raw cashews, soaked for 2 hours and drained

2½ cups unsweetened almond milk

3 tbsp melted palm oil (see note)

½ cup maple syrup

1 tsp pure vanilla extract

½ tsp Himalayan pink salt, plus a pinch

10 Medjool dates, pitted and soaked for 30 minutes

1 Place a shallow glass baking dish in the freezer for at least 1 hour.

2 In a high-speed blender, combine the cashews, almond milk, oil, maple syrup, vanilla, and a pinch of salt. Blend until creamy. Pour the mixture into the chilled glass baking dish.

3 In a food processor, combine the dates and ½ teaspoon salt. Blend until smooth, adding a little almond milk if needed to achieve a creamy consistency.

4 Using a spatula or butter knife, swirl the date mixture into the cashew mixture. Cover and freeze overnight. Set out for 20 minutes prior to scooping. Ice cream can be stored in the freezer for up to 1 week but is best when fresh.

note

Be sure to use sustainably sourced palm oil. If unavailable, coconut oil can be used instead.

chocolate chickpea ice cream

Ice cream and chickpeas may sound like an unlikely combo, but we bet you'll be pleasantly surprised by this rich and creamy, protein-packed treat. It's an excellent vegan dessert loved by kids and parents alike!

Yield **4 servings**	Prep Time **15 minutes, plus overnight freeze**	Cook Time **None**	80:20

½ cup unsweetened almond milk

4 ripe bananas, frozen

4 Medjool dates, pitted and soaked for 30 minutes

½ cup cooked chickpeas

¾ cup unsweetened sunflower seed butter

¼ cup raw cacao powder

1 tsp pure vanilla extract

Pinch of Himalayan pink salt

Cacao nibs or dairy-free mini chocolate chips, for topping

1 Place a shallow glass baking dish in the freezer for at least 1 hour.

2 In a high-speed blender, combine the almond milk, bananas, dates, chickpeas, sunflower seed butter, cacao powder, vanilla, and salt. Blend on medium-low speed until smooth and creamy, using the tamper to push down the mixture if necessary. Keep the setting on low to get the proper consistency. If needed, add an extra splash of almond milk to achieve a smooth, creamy texture.

3 Pour the mixture into the chilled glass baking dish, cover, and freeze overnight. Remove from the freezer 20 minutes prior to scooping. Serve topped with cacao nibs or chocolate chips. Ice cream can be kept in the freezer for up to 1 week.

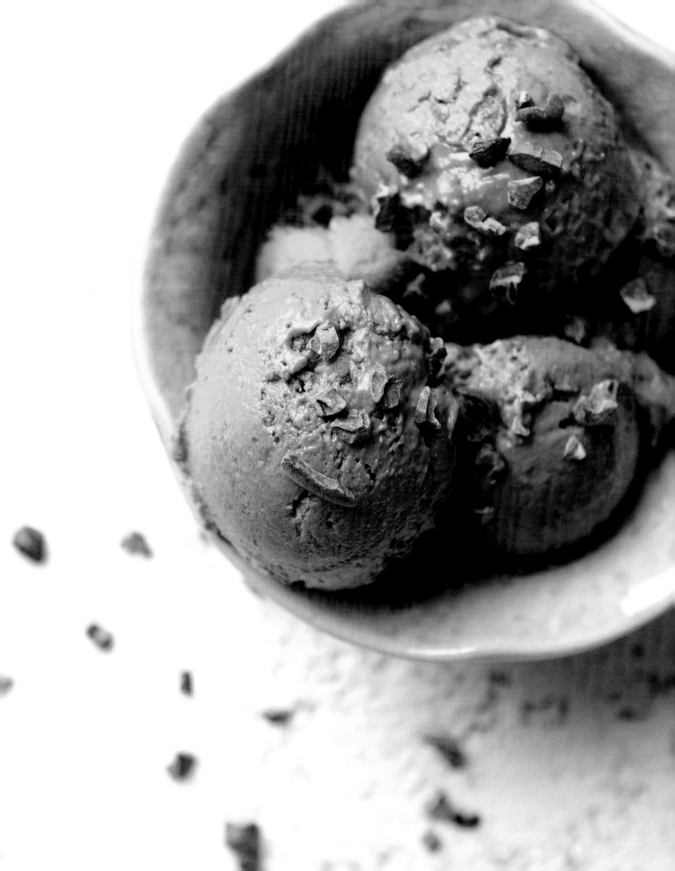

beverages & elixirs

homemade plant-based milks.............................230

carob hot cocoa 232

dandelion detox koffee....................................233

matcha green tea latte.....................................233

turmeric tonic latte 235

vegan white russian 236

lemon ginger switchel 237

jalapeño cilantro mezcal margarita 238

homemade plant-based milks

Once you've made your own homemade, plant-based milk, which is creamy and frothy without all the fillers, it's nearly impossible to go back to the store-bought varieties. Here we've included all our personal favorites, which we like to rotate on a regular basis to provide for optimal nutrient diversity.

CASHEW MILK

Yield **4 cups**
Prep Time **3 minutes, plus overnight soak**
Cook Time **None**

 CLEANSE

1 cup raw cashews, soaked overnight and drained

4 cups filtered water

Pinch of Himalayan pink salt

In a high-speed blender, combine the soaked cashews, filtered water, salt, and any optional flavor additions. Blend until smooth and creamy. Store in the refrigerator for up to 5 days.

ALMOND MILK

Yield **4 cups**
Prep Time **5 minutes, plus overnight soak**
Cook Time **None**

 CLEANSE

1 cup raw almonds, soaked overnight and drained

4 cups filtered water

Pinch of Himalayan pink salt

1 In a high-speed blender, blend the almonds and filtered water on high for 2 minutes. Strain through a nut milk bag, and discard the leftover pulp.

2 Rinse the blender cup, and pour in the strained nut milk. Add the salt and any optional flavor additions. Blend until smooth. Store in the refrigerator for up to 5 days.

BRAZIL NUT MILK

Yield **4 cups**
Prep Time **5 minutes, plus overnight soak**
Cook Time **None**

 CLEANSE

1 cup raw Brazil nuts, soaked overnight and drained

4 cups filtered water

Pinch of Himalayan pink salt

1 In a high-speed blender, blend the soaked nuts and filtered water on high for 2 minutes. Strain through a nut milk bag, and discard the leftover pulp.

2 Rinse the blender cup, and pour in the strained nut milk. Add the salt and any optional flavor additions. Blend until smooth. Store in the refrigerator for up to 5 days.

OAT MILK

Yield **5 cups**
Prep Time **5 minutes, plus 15-minute soak**
Cook Time **None**

 80:20

4 cups filtered water

Pinch of Himalayan pink salt

3 ice cubes

1 cup gluten-free oats, soaked for 15 minutes, drained, and rinsed

1   In a high-speed blender, combine the filtered water, salt, and any optional flavor additions. Blend until creamy. Add the ice cubes and oats, and blend again for 15 seconds, being careful not to warm the liquid or overblend.

2   Place a mesh sieve over a wide-mouth glass jar. Strain the oat milk through the sieve, and discard any leftover oat pulp. Store in the refrigerator for up to 5 days.

HEMP MILK

Yield **3 cups**
Prep Time **3 minutes**
Cook Time **None**

 CLEANSE

3 cups filtered water

1 cup hemp seeds

Pinch of Himalayan pink salt

In a high-speed blender, combine the filtered water, hemp seeds, salt, and any optional flavor additions. Blend until smooth and creamy. Store in the refrigerator for up to 5 days.

COCONUT MILK

Yield **4 cups**
Prep Time **3 minutes**
Cook Time **None**

 CLEANSE

4 cups filtered water

2 cups shredded coconut

Pinch of Himalayan pink salt

1   In a high-speed blender, blend the filtered water and shredded coconut on high for 2 minutes. Strain coconut milk through a nut milk bag.

2   Rinse the blender cup, and pour in the strained coconut milk. Add the salt and any optional flavor additions, and blend to combine. Store in the refrigerator for up to 5 days.

variations

For sweeter flavor, add 1–2 Medjool dates and 2 teaspoons pure vanilla extract.

For strawberry milk, add 2 cups fresh strawberries and blend to combine (80:20 only).

For cinnamon milk, add 1 teaspoon ground cinnamon.

For chocolate milk, add 1–2 tablespoons cacao powder (80:20 only).

carob hot cocoa
WITH COCONUT WHIPPED CREAM

This recipe was contributed by our right-hand woman, Mel, who, like us, knows that some days just call for hot cocoa! In Colorado, when the snow is coming down and the kids are out sledding and building snow forts, this is our go-to warming treat. Top it with coconut whipped cream, and your kiddos will never miss the chemical-laden boxed hot cocoa.

Yield **2–4 servings**	Prep Time **15 minutes**	Cook Time **5 minutes**	CLEANSE

For the whipped cream (optional)

1 (13.5oz) can full-fat coconut milk, refrigerated overnight

1½ tbsp honey

1½ tsp pure vanilla extract

For the cocoa

4 cups **Almond Milk** (page 230) or favorite nut milk of choice

4 tbsp roasted carob powder

½ tsp vanilla powder

Pinch of Himalayan pink salt

2 tbsp honey, or 1–2 packets stevia (optional)

Dash or cayenne pepper or ground cinnamon

1 To make the whipped cream, if using, carefully open the can of refrigerated coconut milk. Keeping the can level, scrape out the thick, waxy top layer of coconut cream, and place in a medium bowl. Save the leftover coconut water from the can for another use. (We like to use it in our green smoothies.) Using a mixer on high speed, whip the coconut cream for 3 minutes or until it becomes light and fluffy. Add the honey and vanilla, and beat for 2 minutes more. Transfer to an airtight container, and refrigerate until ready to use.

2 To make the cocoa, in a medium saucepan, warm the almond milk, carob powder, vanilla powder, and salt over medium-high heat, whisking to break up any clumps. Keep stirring until hot, about 1 to 2 minutes, making sure not to let it boil. Add honey or stevia (if using), stir again, and pour into mugs. Top with the coconut whipped cream, if using, and a dash of cayenne or cinnamon.

dandelion detox koffee

Giving up caffeine can be hard! That's why we created this detox-promoting, coffee-flavored alternative. Start by mixing this with regular coffee, and gradually eliminate regular coffee altogether. When you're free from the artificial energy of caffeine, you'll be amazed at how much energy you have naturally!

Yield **4 servings**	Prep Time **5 minutes**	Cook Time **15 minutes**	CLEANSE

6 cups water

2 tbsp roasted chicory root, finely ground

2 tbsp dandelion root, finely ground

¼ tsp ground cinnamon

1–2 vanilla beans, chopped into pieces, or ¼–½ tsp vanilla powder

Stevia (optional), to taste

Nut milk of choice (optional), steamed and frothed

1. In a 2-quart saucepan, combine the water, chicory root, dandelion root, cinnamon, and vanilla beans. Bring to a boil and then reduce heat to medium-low and simmer for 10 to 15 minutes.

2. Pour the mixture through a fine mesh strainer to remove the grounds. Serve with a few drops of stevia and steamed nut milk, if desired.

matcha green tea latte

This is one of Jo's favorites when she's not cleansing. Matcha, a green tea variety that's full of antioxidants, is known to boost metabolism, improve concentration, and deliver sustained energy without the jitters.

Yield **1 serving**	Prep Time **1 minute**	Cook Time **5 minutes**	80:20

¼ cup water

1 tsp matcha powder (The Tea Spot brand recommended)

¾ cup **Almond Milk** (page 230)

Stevia or honey, to taste (use stevia for low sugar)

In a small saucepan, bring the water to a boil and then whisk in the matcha powder. When the powder has dissolved, whisk in the almond milk and continue to heat on low until warmed. Sweeten to taste with stevia or honey.

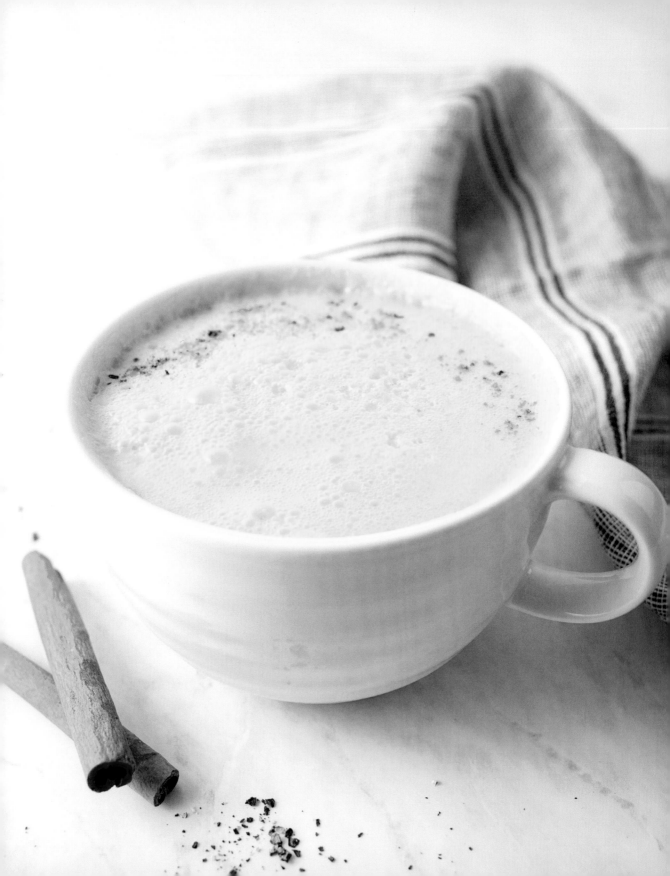

turmeric tonic latte

This is one of our all-time favorite herbal teas. Packed with turmeric, the inflammation-fighting spice, this latte makes a robust and creamy treat while on the Conscious Cleanse.

Yield **1 serving**	Prep Time **5 minutes**	Cook Time **5 minutes**	CLEANSE

1 cup **Coconut Milk** (page 231)

1 rounded tsp minced fresh turmeric

½ rounded tsp minced fresh ginger

¼ tsp freshly ground black pepper

1 cinnamon stick

1 tsp coconut oil

1 tbsp honey, or 1 packet stevia (optional; use stevia for low sugar)

1 In a small saucepan, heat the coconut milk, turmeric, ginger, pepper, cinnamon stick, and coconut oil over medium heat, whisking frequently for 4 minutes or until hot.

2 Remove the cinnamon stick, and transfer the mixture to a high-speed blender. Add honey or stevia, if using, and blend on high for 1 to 2 minutes or until frothy. Pour into a mug with the cinnamon stick, and serve.

tip

Be careful when blending hot liquids. Always use the blender lid and cap, and as an extra precaution, we like to place a kitchen towel over the top, too.

note

We love this tea so much, we partnered with The Tea Spot to craft our very own tea line. Try their Organic Turmeric Tonic tea blend in place of the fresh spices called for here.

vegan white russian

This is a festive family favorite in Jules' household—especially around the holidays! Keeping this dairy-free is easy. Just swap out the half-and-half for a creamy, homemade nut or oat milk, and this is one dreamy and delicious cocktail that won't leave you feeling phlegmy.

Yield **1 serving**	Prep Time **5 minutes**	Cook Time **None**	80:20

2 oz vodka

2 tbsp coffee liqueur (Kahlúa brand recommended)

¼ cup **Cashew Milk** (page 230) or **Oat Milk** (page 231)

In a cocktail shaker, combine the vodka, coffee liqueur, and cashew or oat milk. Add 6 ice cubes, seal the lid, and shake well. Strain into an ice-filled old-fashioned glass.

lemon ginger switchel

If you love a Moscow Mule but don't love all the sugar packed into a bottle of ginger beer, you're going to love this variation. Made with fresh-pressed lemon and ginger, this is the perfect refreshing cocktail or mocktail, delicious with or without the alcohol.

Yield **2 quarts**	Prep Time **5 minutes**	Cook Time **25 minutes**	80:20

1 cup roughly chopped fresh ginger

¾ cup maple syrup or honey

½ cup apple cider vinegar

⅔ cup freshly squeezed lemon juice

Gin or vodka (optional), to serve

1 Place the ginger in a 2-quart saucepan, and add filtered water until the pan is two-thirds full. Bring to a boil over high heat, and boil for about 2 minutes. Remove from heat, cover, and let the ginger steep for 20 minutes.

2 In a 2-quart pitcher or Mason jar, combine the maple syrup or honey, vinegar, and lemon juice. Strain the ginger-infused water into the pitcher, discarding the ginger pieces. Stir to mix all ingredients well.

3 Serve over ice, with 1 to 2 ounces of gin or vodka per serving, if using.

jalapeño cilantro mezcal margarita

If we're going to indulge in a cocktail, a high-quality 100 percent agave tequila is usually our go-to because it's the cleanest choice. Mezcal, known for its signature smoky flavor, is tequila's favorite cousin. Here we've created a cocktail that delivers a fiesta of flavor—smoky, tart, and just a little sweet—with a perfect kick of heat from the jalapeño.

Yield **1 serving**	Prep Time **5 minutes**	Cook Time **None**	80:20

Juice of 2 limes, divided

1–2 jalapeño slices, plus more to garnish

2 tbsp fresh cilantro leaves, plus more to garnish

Juice of ½ grapefruit

2 oz mezcal

1 tsp agave nectar (optional, omit for low sugar)

Pineapple slice (optional), to garnish

1 Pour ¼ cup lime juice into a cocktail shaker. Add the jalapeño and cilantro. Muddle the jalapeño and cilantro in the lime juice.

2 Add the grapefruit juice, mezcal, remaining lime juice, agave, if using, and several ice cubes. Shake to mix the ingredients thoroughly.

3 Fill your favorite glass with ice, and strain the margarita into the glass. Garnish with a slice of pineapple, if using, a sprig of cilantro, or a slice of jalapeño for extra spice. Enjoy!

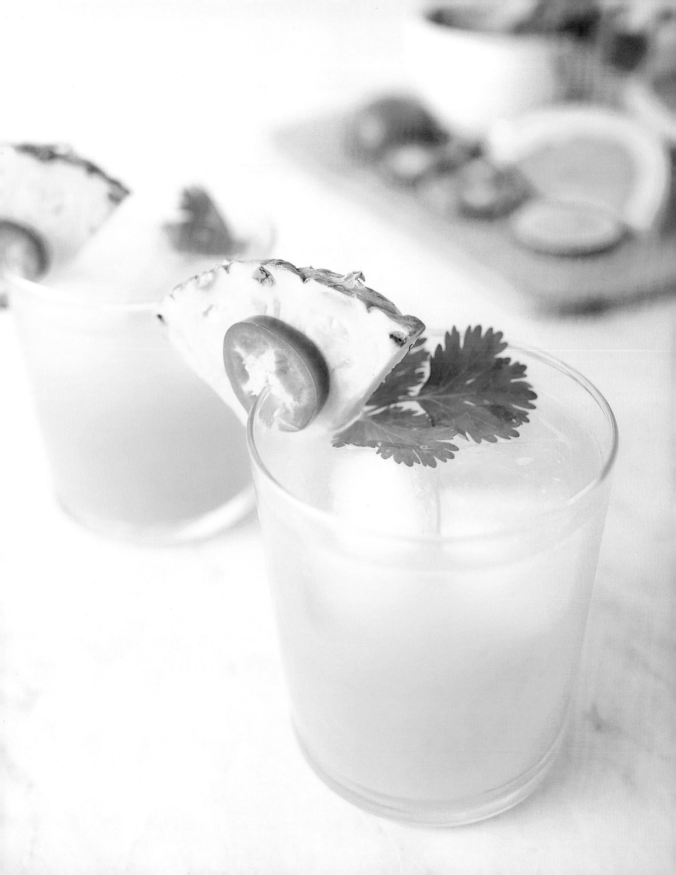

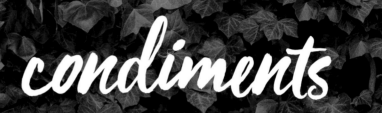

condiments

vegan kimchi.. 242

cashew feta 243

no-mato marinara 244

egg-free avocado mayo 245

green tzatziki sauce 245

homemade pestos 246

vegan kimchi

Want to make your gut happy? Enjoy a tablespoon or two of this probiotic-rich fermented cabbage. Having a healthy and balanced microbiome is crucial for vibrant health and is linked to lowering the incidence of allergies, chronic illness, autoimmune disease, heart disease, eczema, and depression, just to name a few.

| Yield **4–6 cups** | Prep Time **20 minutes, plus 5 days to ferment** | Cook Time **None** | CLEANSE |

1 medium head green cabbage, quartered and cored

5 carrots, peeled

6 red radishes, or 1 small daikon radish

3 Hakurei turnips

½ cup sliced scallions

2½ tsp Himalayan pink salt

3-in piece fresh ginger, peeled and coarsely chopped

8 cloves garlic

2 tbsp red pepper flakes

1 In a food processor fitted with the shredder blade, shred the cabbage, carrots, radishes, and turnips. Transfer to a large bowl, and add the scallions and salt. Toss to combine.

2 Change food processor blade to the s-blade and blend the ginger, garlic, and red pepper flakes until finely ground. Scrape the sides and blend again. Add the mixture to the vegetables, and use your hands to mix thoroughly. Continue mixing and massaging the vegetables for a few minutes until they become juicy and start to soften.

3 Add a handful of vegetables each to two wide-mouth, quart-size canning jars, and pound down firmly with your fist or a muddler to release any air pockets. Repeat with remaining vegetables, a handful at a time, then divide any remaining liquid from the bowl between the jars.

4 The vegetables should be submerged below the liquid. If they aren't, push the vegetables down until the liquid rises. Press any pieces of cabbage down from the sides of the jars so they are submerged as well.

5 Fill two smaller jars or bottles with water, and place them on the surface of the vegetables as a weight to keep them below the liquid.

6 Cover both jars with tight-fitting lids to keep any particles out. Place in a cool, well-ventilated area. Ferment for at least 5 to 7 days or for up to 10 days or longer.

7 After 5 days, taste the kimchi and then again every day until the flavor is to your liking. To store, cover the jars with a lid and refrigerate. The kimchi will keep for months, and the flavor will continue to develop and strengthen. Don't worry if the veggies soften—it is all just part of the process.

cashew feta

This vegan, plant-based "cheese" is a delicious alternative to regular feta, perfect while on the Conscious Cleanse. And really, who needs dairy when you have cashews?!

Yield **1 cup**	Prep Time **10 minutes, plus 1-hour soak**	Cook Time **None**	**LS** CLEANSE

1 cup raw cashews, soaked for 1 hour and drained

2 tsp freshly squeezed lemon juice

½ tsp Himalayan pink salt

Freshly ground black pepper, to taste

In a food processor, combine all ingredients and pulse for about 10 seconds. If needed, add 1 tablespoon water to make creamier, and pulse again. Store in an airtight container for up to 1 week.

variation

To make a spreadable cashew cheese, add an additional ¼ cup water and process for 2 to 4 minutes or until completely smooth. Adjust the salt and pepper to taste.

no-mato marinara

Eliminating nightshades on the Conscious Cleanse can be challenging. Life without tomatoes takes some getting used to, as Jules will attest! Enter "no-mato" sauce—that is, marinara sauce made without tomatoes. We love this over zucchini noodles with our Plant-Powered Not-Meat Balls or even on top of roasted veggies. Top with some goat cheese when not cleansing for an extra-creamy treat!

Yield **2 cups**	Prep Time **20 minutes**	Cook Time **75 minutes**	CLEANSE

1 small beet

1 tbsp olive oil

1 medium white onion, diced

1 cup diced carrots

1 cup cubed summer squash

2–4 cloves garlic, crushed

2 tbsp chopped fresh basil

1½ tbsp dried Italian seasoning

1 tbsp freshly squeezed lemon juice

4 tbsp apple cider vinegar

1½ tsp Himalayan pink salt

1 Preheat the oven to 375°F. Rinse the beet and trim off the leafy top. Wrap loosely in foil, and place in the oven. Roast for 1 hour or until soft. Remove from the oven, take off foil, and set aside to cool. When cool enough to handle, cut off the top and peel the skin. (You should be able to do this easily with your fingers.) Cut into quarters, and set aside.

2 In a medium saucepan, heat the oil over medium-high heat. Add the onion and carrots, and sauté for 4 minutes or until the onions become translucent.

3 In a high-speed blender, combine the roasted beet, cooked onion and carrots, squash, garlic, basil, Italian seasoning, lemon juice, vinegar, and salt. Blend until smooth.

4 Transfer the blended ingredients to a saucepan, and simmer for 15 minutes. Store in a glass container in the refrigerator for 7 days.

egg-free avocado mayo

This is a terrific alternative to egg-based mayonnaise, delivering the creaminess of mayo with the added benefits of our favorite superfruit, avocado. It's delicious on our Chipotle Lime Lentil Burger or as a dip.

Yield **1 cup**	Prep Time **5 minutes**	Cook Time **None**	CLEANSE

1 avocado, cubed

1 tbsp Dijon mustard

2 tbsp freshly squeezed lemon juice

1 clove garlic

2 tbsp olive oil

¼ tsp Himalayan pink salt

¼ tsp freshly ground black pepper

1 In a food processor, combine all ingredients. Blend until smooth.

2 Refrigerate in a glass jar for up to 4 days. If a brown layer forms on top, simply scrape it off before eating.

green tzatziki sauce

A dairy-free spin on tzatziki, which is usually made with Greek yogurt, this light and refreshing sauce is delicious on sandwiches, like our Lamb Gyro Lettuce Wrap, or served as a dip with a mezze spread.

Yield **1½ cups**	Prep Time **15 minutes, plus overnight soak**	Cook Time **None**	CLEANSE

½ cup macadamia nuts, soaked overnight and drained

½ cup water

2 tbsp finely chopped fresh dill

1 clove garlic

1½ tsp freshly squeezed lemon juice

1½ tsp lemon zest

½ tsp Himalayan pink salt

¼ cup peeled and finely diced English cucumber

In a high-speed blender, combine the macadamia nuts, water, dill, garlic, lemon juice, zest, and salt. Blend on high until smooth and creamy. Transfer to a bowl and stir in the cucumber.

homemade pestos

To say that we love pesto would be an understatement. Garden fresh and so versatile, pesto is perfect to keep on hand for a quick dinner with zucchini noodles, as a dip with crudité, or for topping our Quinoa Flatbread Pizza. Traditional pesto is made with pine nuts and basil, but we like to switch it up based on what we have available. Swap in walnuts or sunflower seeds in place of pine nuts. Add in any dark leafy greens for a slightly different variation—use those "double agents," like beet greens and carrot tops! Pesto also freezes well, so you can freeze it in an ice cube tray for easy defrosting.

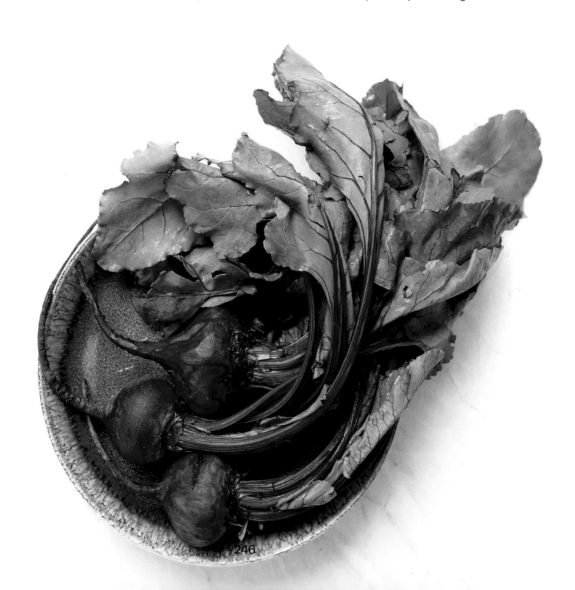

ARUGULA PESTO

Yield **1 cup**
Prep Time **10 minutes**
Cook Time **None**

 CLEANSE

1 clove garlic

1 cup arugula, packed

½ cup fresh basil, packed

Juice of ½ lemon (about 1 tbsp)

¼ cup pine nuts

½ tsp Himalayan pink salt

Freshly ground black pepper, to taste

¼ cup olive oil

In a high-speed blender or food processor, pulse the garlic until minced, then scrape down the sides. Add the arugula, basil, lemon juice, pine nuts, salt, and pepper. Blend until smooth and creamy. While the food processor is running, drizzle in the oil until fully emulsified.

BEET GREEN PESTO

Yield **1 cup**
Prep Time **10 minutes**
Cook Time **None**

 CLEANSE

1 clove garlic

1½ cups beet greens, packed

½ cup fresh basil, packed

Juice of ½ lemon (about 1 tbsp)

¼ cup walnuts

½ tsp Himalayan pink salt

Freshly ground black pepper, to taste

¼ cup olive oil

In a high-speed blender or food processor, process the garlic until minced, then scrape down the sides. Add the beet greens, basil, lemon juice, walnuts, salt, and pepper, and process until smooth and creamy. With the food processor running, drizzle in the oil until fully emulsified.

CARROT TOP PESTO

Yield **1 cup**
Prep Time **10 minutes**
Cook Time **None**

 CLEANSE

1 clove garlic

Greens from 1 bunch organic carrots, thoroughly washed

¼ cup raw almonds or sunflower seeds, soaked for 4 hours, drained and rinsed

⅓ cup olive oil

¼ tsp Himalayan pink salt

Freshly ground black pepper, to taste

In a high-speed blender or food processor, process the garlic until minced, then scrape down the sides. Add the carrot greens and almonds or sunflower seeds. Pulse a few times to break up the ingredients. With the food processor running, slowly drizzle in the oil until the mixture is emulsified but still has some texture. Add salt and pepper, and pulse once more.

variation

What about cheese? If you love a cheesy pesto, add 1 tablespoon nutritional yeast (when not cleansing) for a boost of B vitamins and a creamier, cheesier pesto.

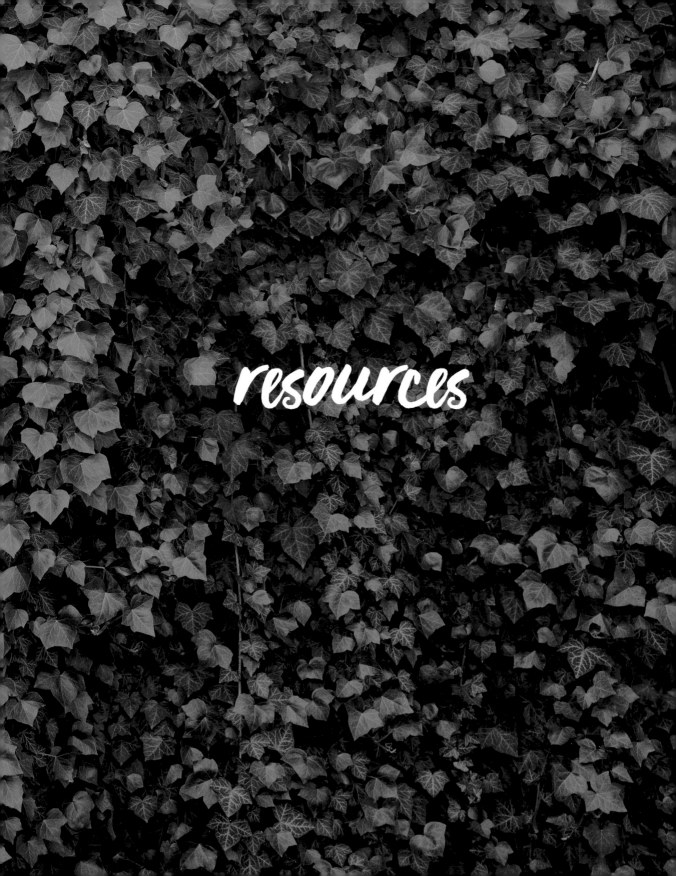

brands we love and trust

365 Everyday Value: sugar-free Dijon mustard

Anthony's Goods: almond flour, cassava flour, arrow-root powder, spirulina powder

Artisana Organics: organic raw nut butters and tahini

Bob's Red Mill: organic gluten-free oats, chickpea flour, oat flour

Bragg's: apple cider vinegar

Califia Farms: unsweetened almond milk

Coconut Secret: coconut aminos

Doctor in the Kitchen: Flackers (flaxseed crackers)

Eden Foods: organic beans, ume plum vinegar, seaweed gomasio

Enjoy Life: dairy-free chocolate chips

Food for Life: gluten-free rice millet bread

Frontier Co-Op: herbs and spices

Gemini Superfoods: tiger nut flour

Green & Black's: 88 percent organic dark chocolate

Imagine: organic broths

Inner Ēco: fresh young coconut meat purée (frozen smoothie packs)

JicaTortillas: jicama tortillas

Kasandrinos: organic extra virgin olive oil, balsamic vinegar, red wine vinegar

Kim and Jake's: gluten-free bread

Lakanto: classic monk fruit sweetener

Manitoba Harvest: organic hemp hearts

Native Forest: organic full-fat canned coconut milk and coconut cream

Navitas Organics: organic maca, raw cacao powder, açai powder, cacao butter

Nutiva: organic coconut oil, chia seeds

Ozuké: fermented foods

Pacific Foods: organic broths

Pamela's: cassava four

Picaflor: sriracha sauce

Pure Mountain Botanicals: liquid stevia

Red Boat: sugar-free fish sauce

Sir Kensington's: egg-free chickpea vegan mayo

South River: chickpea miso

SweetLeaf: organic powdered stevia

Thai Kitchen: sugar-free chili paste, organic full-fat canned coconut milk

The Tea Spot: premium organic whole leaf tea

Wild Planet: canned sardines

meal plans

These 7-day meal plans demonstrate how you might utilize the guidance of our different Conscious Cleanse tracks. Remember, there are no hard-and-fast rules to follow except to commit to showing up and doing your best. We've taken our two most popular tracks—Meat Lover/Low Sugar and Plant Powered—to show you how you might approach meal planning while on the Conscious Cleanse. Please realize that we do not expect you to cook breakfast, lunch, and dinner every day. Make extra at dinnertime, and enjoy the leftovers for lunch the next day. Batch cook on the weekends to prepare dips, snacks, sauces, and nongluten grains ahead of time. When in doubt, reach for fresh fruit or raw veggies while you figure out what else to eat.

MEAT LOVER / LOW SUGAR PLAN

Day 1

BREAKFAST: Jo's Super Green Smoothie (p44)

LUNCH: Ginger Salmon Bowl (p148)

DINNER: Grilled Chicken (p137) with Simple Kale Salad (p83)

SNACK: Roasted Garlic Cauliflower Hummus (p181) with celery and carrot sticks

Day 2

BREAKFAST: Cran-Pear Smoothie (p46)

LUNCH: Simple Kale Salad (p83)

DINNER: Greek Wedge Salad with Braised Lamb (p86)

SNACK: Spinach Artichoke Dip (p188) with cucumber slices

Day 3

BREAKFAST: Apple Pie Smoothie (p47)

LUNCH: Lamb Gyro Lettuce Wrap (p129)

DINNER: Salt & Pepper Snapper (p147) with Jules' Salad of Abundance (p84)

SNACK: Curry Roasted Cashews (p195)

Day 4

BREAKFAST: Mint Green Sweetie Smoothie (p53)

LUNCH: Mason Jar Chopped Salad (p97)

DINNER: Ginger Scallion Turkey Burger (p142) with Parsnip Fries (p197)

SNACK: Carob Chia Pudding (p204)

Day 5

BREAKFAST: Power-Up Protein Smoothie (p56)

LUNCH: Mediterranean Lettuce Wrap (p172)

DINNER: Bison Bolognese with Zucchini Noodles (p132)

SNACK: Golden Flaxseed Crackers (p192)

Day 6 (PURIFICATION)

BREAKFAST: Lemon Lime Cucumber Cooler (p57)

LUNCH: Purification Soup (p116)

DINNER: Clean & Simple Stir-Fry (p161)

SNACK: Jo's Super Green Smoothie (p44)

Day 7 (PURIFICATION)

BREAKFAST: Green Ollie Smoothie (p46)

LUNCH: Roasted Rainbow Veggies (p177)

DINNER: Golden Soup (p115) with 4 oz Ginger Salmon (p148)

SNACK: Spicy Greens Juice (p59)

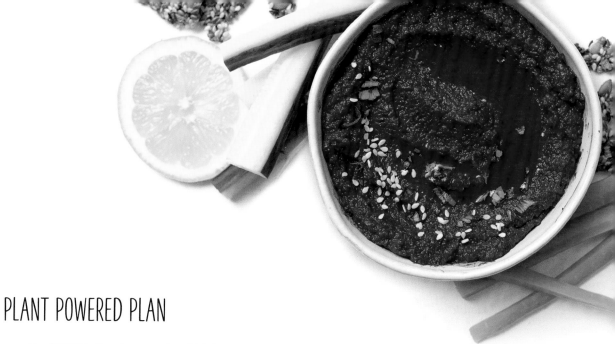

PLANT POWERED PLAN

Day 1

BREAKFAST: Jules' Go-To Green Juice (p59)

LUNCH: Jules' Salad of Abundance (p84)

DINNER: Healing Vegetable Congee (p112)

SNACK: The Great Eliminator (p49)

Day 2

BREAKFAST: Natural Bzzz Green Smoothie (p43)

LUNCH: Veggie Sushi Hand Roll (p173)

DINNER: Chipotle Lime Lentil Burger (p164) with Simple Kale Salad (p83)

SNACK: Garlicky Dill Dip (p180) with celery and carrot sticks

Day 3

BREAKFAST: Spicy Greens Juice (p59)

LUNCH: Mason Jar Chopped Salad (p97)

DINNER: Veggie Kelp Noodle Pho (p113)

SNACK: Spirulina Smoothie (p49)

Day 4

BREAKFAST: "Get the Glow" Green Smoothie (p48)

LUNCH: Winter Roasted Veggie Salad (p99)

DINNER: Vegan Chickpea Curry (p168)

SNACK: Beet Hummus (p182) with celery and carrot sticks

Day 5

BREAKFAST: Lemon Blueberry Smoothie (p54)

LUNCH: Warm Kale & Beet Rice Salad (p98)

DINNER: Millet Vibrancy Bowl (p157)

SNACK: Super Seaweed Crackers (p193) and Simple Guacamole (p184)

Day 6
(PURIFICATION)

BREAKFAST: Heavy Metals Be Gone Juice (p58)

LUNCH: Purification Soup (p116)

DINNER: Clean & Simple Stir-Fry (p161)

SNACK: Cardio Booster Juice (p58)

Day 7
(PURIFICATION)

BREAKFAST: Green Ollie Smoothie (p46)

LUNCH: Roasted Rainbow Veggies (p177)

DINNER: Cleansing Ginger Beet Soup (p110)

SNACK: Jo's Super Green Smoothie (p44)

index

A

Ahi Tuna Poke Bowl 146
allergens, elimination of 17
Almond Milk 230
Apple Cider Vinaigrette 92
Apple Pie Smoothie 47
Arugula Pesto 171, 247
Autumn Wild Rice Salad 102

B

Baked Oatmeal Cups 66
beets
    Beet Green Pesto 247
    Beet Hummus 182
    Cleansing Ginger Beet Soup 110
    Warm Kale & Beet Rice Salad 98
Bison Bolognese with Zucchini
    Noodles 132
Bison Broccoli Stir-Fry 130
blueberries
    Blueberry Hemp Bites 69
    Lemon Blueberry Smoothie 54
BPA-free products 19
Brazil Nut Milk 230
Breakfast Niçoise Salad 74
broccoli, Bison Broccoli Stir-Fry 130
buddy system 33
Butter Lettuce Salad with Lime Fig
    Dressing 95
butternut squash
    Butternut Curry Sauce 145
    Slow Cooker Butternut Lentil Soup
    117

C

cabbage, Roasted Cabbage 165
Cardio Booster Juice 58
Carob Avocado Frosting 209
Carob Chia Pudding 204

Carob Hazelnut Cheesecake 224
Carob Hot Cocoa with Coconut
    Whipped Cream 232
carrots
    Carrot Cake in a Bowl 47
    Carrot Top Pesto 247
    Carrot Top Pesto Salad 105
    No-Bake Mini Carrot Cake Bites
    218
    Steamed Sea Bass with Carrots
    and Bok Choy 150
cashews 36
    Cashew Chicken Stir-Fry 135
    Cashew Cupcakes with Fresh
    Raspberry Frosting 207
    Cashew Feta 243
    Cashew Milk 230
    Curry Roasted Cashews 195
    Herb & Cashew Crusted Chicken
    with Lemony Arugula 133
cauliflower
    Fried Cauliflower Rice 174
    Roasted Garlic Cauliflower
    Hummus 181
Celery Toast 163
Chia Berry Jam 72
chicken
    Cashew Chicken Stir-Fry 135
    Chicken Bone Broth 108
    Curry Chicken Salad 139
    Dry Rub Chicken Wings 138
    Grilled Chicken with Tomato-Free
    BBQ Sauce 137
    Herb & Cashew Crusted Chicken
    with Lemony Arugula 133
    Honey Mustard Chicken Skewers
    134
    Vietnamese Chicken Pho 123
chickpeas 37
    Chickpea Rosemary Flatbread 187
    Chocolate Chickpea Ice Cream
    226
    Roasted Chickpeas 196
    Spicy Kale Caesar with Crunchy
    Chickpeas 87
    Vegan Chickpea Curry 168
Chipotle Lime Lentil Burger 164

Chipotle Lime Salmon with Massaged
    Kale 143
Chocolate Cherry Smoothie 53
Chocolate Chickpea Ice Cream 226
Chocolate Chip Cookie Dough Balls
    217
Chocolate Dessert Hummus 212
Chocolate Tahini Energy Balls 215
Clean & Simple Stir-Fry 161
Cleansing Ginger Beet Soup 110
Coconut Cream Frosting 209
Coconut Glazed Halibut with
    Butternut Curry Sauce 145
Coconut Milk 231
Conscious Cleanse Plate 22
Cran-Pear Smoothie 46
Creamy Vegan Coleslaw 90
Curry Chicken Salad 139
Curry Rice Salad 160
Curry Roasted Cashews 195

D

Dairy-Free Coconut Yogurt with Chia
    Berry Jam 72
Dandelion Detox Koffee 233
digestion 18, 20
dining out 33
Dragon Fruit Smoothie Bowl 51
Dry Rub Chicken Wings 138

E

Easy Weeknight Fish Tacos 153
eating out 33
Egg-Free Avocado Mayo 245
Egg-Free Veggie Scramble 64
80:20 Lifestyle Plan 24–25

F

Fall Harvest Salad with Apple Cider
    Vinaigrette 92
Five-Ingredient Breakfast Cookies 67
Five-Spice Pumpkin Cookies 205
food allergens, elimination of 17
food combinations 20–21
food reintroduction phase 25
Fresh Raspberry Frosting 207
Fried Cauliflower Rice 174
frosting
    Carob Avocado Frosting 209
    Coconut Cream Frosting 209
    Fresh Raspberry Frosting 207
fruit
    Apple Pie Smoothie 47
    Blueberry Hemp Bites 69
    Chia Berry Jam 72
    Chocolate Cherry Smoothie 53
    Cran-Pear Smoothie 46
    Dragon Fruit Smoothie Bowl 51
    Immune Blaster Juice Shot 61
    Lemon Blueberry Smoothie 54
    Lemon Lime Cucumber Cooler 57
    Lime Fig Dressing 95
    Peach Crumble Bars 202
    Zesty Lemon Balls 216

G

Garlicky Dill Dip 180
Garlic Yam Spread 189
"Get the Glow" Green Smoothie 48
getting started 31–39
Ginger Salmon Bowl 148
Ginger Scallion Turkey Burgers 142
Golden Flaxseed Crackers 192
Golden Soup 115
Good Better Best Guide 27
Grain-Free Nutty Granola 70
Great Eliminator, The 49
Greek-Style Braised Lamb 128
Greek Wedge Salad with Braised
    Lamb 86
Green Ollie Smoothie 46
Greensicle Popsicle 213
green smoothie, how to build 42
Green Tahini Dressing 157
Green Tzatziki Sauce 245
Grilled Chicken with Tomato-Free
    BBQ Sauce 137
Gut-Healing Slaw 91

H–I

Healing Vegetable Congee 112
Heavy Metals Be Gone Juice 58
Hemp Milk 231
Hemp Seed Tabbouleh 94
Herb & Cashew Crusted Chicken with
    Lemony Arugula 133
Homemade Pestos 246–47
Homemade Plant-Based Milks
    230–31
homemade staples 19
Honey Mustard Chicken Skewers 134
Honey Mustard Vinaigrette 83

icons explained 39
Immune Blaster Juice Shot 61

J

Jalapeño Cilantro Mezcal Margarita
    238
Jo's Super Green Smoothie 44
Jules' Go-To Green Juice 59
Jules' Salad of Abundance 84

K

kale
    Chipotle Lime Salmon with
        Massaged Kale 143
    Simple Kale Salad with Honey
        Mustard Vinaigrette 83
    Spicy Kale Caesar with Crunchy
        Chickpeas 87
    Warm Kale & Beet Rice Salad 98
kitchen preparation 36–37
    pantry staples 36–37
        beans and legumes 37
        butters, nut and seed 36
        dried fruits 36
        flours 37
        herbs, spices, and extracts 37
        nongluten grains and
            pseudograins 37
        oils and vinegars 36
        raw nuts and seeds 36
        superfoods 37
        sweeteners 36

L

lamb
    Greek-Style Braised Lamb 128
    Greek Wedge Salad with Braised
        Lamb 86
    Lamb Gyro Lettuce Wrap 129
    Slow Cooker Lamb Tagine 126
Lemon Balls 216
Lemon Blueberry Smoothie 54
Lemon Ginger Switchel 237
Lemon Lime Cucumber Cooler 57
Lemon Thyme Vinaigrette 74
lentils 37
    Chipotle Lime Lentil Burger 164
    Slow Cooker Butternut Lentil Soup
        117
Lime Fig Dressing 95
low-sugar plan 34

M

Maple Sage Breakfast Sausage 78
Maple Tahini Dressing 99
Mason Jar Chopped Salad with Red
    Wine Vinaigrette 97
Matcha Green Tea Latte 233
meat lover's plan 34
Mediterranean Lettuce Wrap 172
Mexican Rice Bowl 158
milks (recipes) 230–31
Millet Vibrancy Bowl with Green Tahini
    Dressing 157
Mint Chocolate Chip Smoothie 48
Mint Green Sweetie Smoothie 53
misconceptions 38
Molten Chocolate Cake with Coconut
    Whipped Cream 210

N

Natural Bzzz Green Smoothie 43
Nightshade-Free Turkey Chili 121
No-Bake Mini Carrot Cake Bites 218
No-Mato Marinara 166, 244
nonstarchy vegetables 21

O

oatmeal, Baked Oatmeal Cups 66
Oat Milk 231

P

pantry staples 36–37
    beans and legumes 37
    butters, nut and seed 36
    dried fruits 36
    flours 37
    herbs, spices, and extracts 37
    nongluten grains and
      pseudograins 37
    oils and vinegars 36
    raw nuts and seeds 36
    superfoods 37
    sweeteners 36
Parsnip Fries 197
Peach Crumble Bars 202
pestos (recipes) 171, 246–47
Plant-Powered Not-Meat Balls with
    Zoodles and No-Mato Marinara 166
plant-powered plan 34
Plant-Powered Queso Dip 185
Power-Up Protein Smoothie 56
pumpkin
    Five-Spice Pumpkin Cookies 205
    Pumpkin Fudge 223
pumpkin seeds 36
Purification, preparation for 32
Purification Soup 116

Q–R

quinoa 37
    Quinoa Flatbread Pizza with
      Arugula Pesto 171
    Quinoa Watercress Salad 103

Real-Deal Protein Powders 52
Red Wine Vinaigrette 97
Roasted Cabbage 165
Roasted Chickpeas 196
Roasted Garlic Cauliflower Hummus
    181
Roasted Rainbow Veggies 177

S

Salt & Pepper Snapper 147
Salted Caramel Ice Cream 225
Sardines for Breakfast 75
Sesame Cauli Wings 198
Shrimp Pad Thai 140
Simple Guacamole 184
Simple Kale Salad with Honey
    Mustard Vinaigrette 83
slow cooker 36
Slow Cooker Bison Stew 118
Slow Cooker Butternut Lentil Soup 117
Slow Cooker Lamb Tagine 126
Spicy Greens Juice 59
Spicy Kale Caesar with Crunchy
    Chickpeas 87
spinach
    Spinach Artichoke Dip 188
    Sweet Miso Black Cod with
      Garlicky Spinach 151
Spirulina Smoothie 49
Squashie Pancakes 79
staples, homemade 19
Steamed Sea Bass with Carrots and
    Bok Choy 150
stir-fry
    Bison Broccoli Stir-Fry 130
    Cashew Chicken Stir-Fry 135
    Clean & Simple Stir-Fry 161
    Fried Cauliflower Rice 174
storage containers, glass 36
sugar sensitivity quiz 34
Sunflower Cookies 221
Superfood Bars 190
Superfood Green "Soup" 120
Super Seaweed Crackers 193
supplements 17–18
Sweet Miso Black Cod with Garlicky
    Spinach 151
Sweet Potato Toast 176

T–U

Thai Cucumber Noodle Salad 100
Thai Flank Steak Salad 89
Tomato-Free BBQ Sauce 137
track choices 34
tuna, Ahi Tuna Poke Bowl 146
turkey
    Ginger Scallion Turkey Burgers
      142
    Nightshade-Free Turkey Chili 121
    Turkey Breakfast Skillet 77
Turmeric Tonic Latte 235

V

Vanilla Almond Macaroons with
    Chocolate Drizzle 220
Vanilla Tiger Nut Cupcakes 208
Vegan Chickpea Curry 168
Vegan Kimchi 242
Vegan White Russian 236
Veggie Broth 109
Veggie Egg Muffins 71
Veggie Kelp Noodle Pho 113
Veggie Sushi Hand Roll 173
vibrancy bowl, how to build 156
Vietnamese Chicken Pho 123

W–X–Y–Z

Warm Kale & Beet Rice Salad 98
wild rice 37, 102
Winter Roasted Veggie Salad with
    Maple Tahini Dressing 99

yams, Garlic Yam Spread 189

Zesty Lemon Balls 216
zucchini
    Bison Bolognese with Zucchini
      Noodles 132
    Zucchini Lasagna with Ricotta
      "Cheese" 169

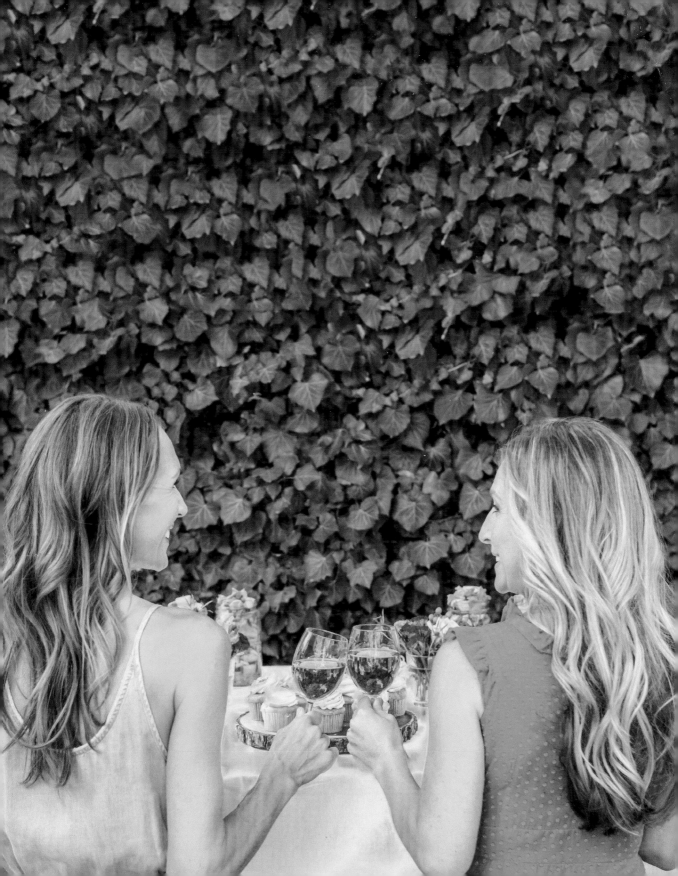

acknowledgments

From Jo and Jules: Thank you, Mel, for your unwavering commitment and steadfast attention to detail. We couldn't have dreamed up a more loyal and loving right-hand woman. To Martha, thank you for the beautiful illustrations you created for this project and for all the creative and technical hats you wear. You amaze us! To Kimba, thank you for joining us in the kitchen and for bringing your culinary creativity and intuition to so many of the recipes in this cookbook. To Julia, thank you for capturing the spirit of this cookbook and for making us laugh with your silly fart jokes. To Ann, you have made what could have been a daunting project, a breeze. Thank you for your easygoing demeanor (even in the face of meeting a deadline during a pandemic), inspiring professionalism, and incredible attention to detail.

From Jo: To my mom, for always believing in me and standing strong in your belief that healing is possible. To my dad, for dreaming big and inspiring me to work hard every day. To my husband, for taking on any recipe challenge, for supporting me unconditionally, and for loving our family fiercely. To my daughter, for being the true light in my life and for making me laugh until my belly hurts.

From Jules: To Enzo, Rocco, and Dax, you are my everything. Being your mom is what fills my heart with joy every single day. To Digger, my favorite dinner companion, had it not been for your encouragement, this cookbook may not have happened. Your whatever-it-takes willingness and unwavering support are the glue that holds our family together. I love you. To Jo, our shared belief in the body's ability to heal is what brought us together. Our differences have created a wide-open, sacred space for people to realize that healing. I'm forever grateful for you and our cocreation. To my amazing family, thank you for listening and helping me navigate this crazy thing called life. I would not be where I am today without your love, support, and friendship. CTM, my sweet friend, thank you for enthusiastically testing nearly every recipe I sent your way. And to the countless teachers, healers, and mentors who have walked before me, thank you for sharing your wisdom and grace with me.

about the authors

Julie (Jules) Peláez is the cofounder of the Conscious Cleanse and a board-certified Holistic Health Coach. For more than 15 years, Jules has championed the health benefits of cleansing the body through eating a living-food, plant-based diet. Jules teaches that food is never just about food—it's a gateway to self-discovery and has the power to create a ripple effect in the rest of your life. A certified yoga teacher and lifelong learner, Jules lives with her husband and three children in the Boulder, Colorado, area.

Jo Schaalman was a state champion gymnast, a nationally ranked diver, and a diving coach. While prepping for medical school, she was T-boned by a semitruck during a cross-country bike tour. As a result of the accident, Jo was told that she wouldn't live a normal life, let alone become a doctor. Her recovery process was both physically and emotionally grueling, but through her own healing, she was able to unlock some universal healing principles that could not only help her, but other people as well. These discoveries became key foundations of the Conscious Cleanse. Because of her experience, Jo is driven to help people who think healing is out of their reach. Although she never became a doctor, Jo has been able to fulfill her lifelong mission of helping people heal. Jo lives in Boulder, Colorado, with her husband and two kids.